YOGA FOR WOMEN

This book on Yoga is designed exclusively for women. Its aim is to show women how Yoga can improve the figure, reduce weight, increase vitality and help them to enjoy life to the full.

The authors claim that if their instructions are followed, women can become better looking, not only by improving their health, but through the development of a more positive interest in life and in dealing with their own physical and mental problems. Like most teachers of Yoga, Nancy Phelan knows cases of women who have astonished everyone, including themselves, by exchanging a drawn and harassed, middle-aged look for a youthful, vital one by discarding stiffness and tension for suppleness, slimness, serenity and poise.

Nancy Phelan and Michael Volin

YOGA FOR WOMEN

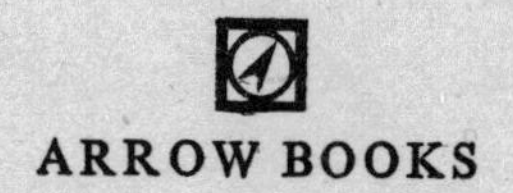

Arrow Books Limited
17–21 Conway Street, London W1P 5HL

An imprint of the Hutchinson Publishing Group

London Melbourne Sydney
Auckland Johannesburg and agencies
throughout the world

First published by Stanley Paul 1963
Arrow edition 1965
Reprinted 1967, 1968
Second edition 1970
Reprinted 1971 (twice), 1972, 1973, 1974, 1978, and 1981

Made and printed in Great Britain
by The Anchor Press Ltd
Tiptree, Essex

ISBN 0 09 916990 8

To
WIN EVERETT

in appreciation
of untiring service
to Michael Volin's
Yoga School, Sydney

Acknowledgements

All the photographs in this book were taken at the London Re-orientation Yoga Centre. We are grateful to both instructors and pupils for their help and co-operation in showing that yoga can be practised by women of any age.

Contents

Asanas are given with English names throughout the book, with the exception of *Savasana* (Position of Complete Rest), *Uddiyana* (stomach contractions), *Nauli* (separation of recti muscles, *Yoga-mudra* (symbol of Yoga) and *Aswini-mudra* (contraction of anus muscles), in all of which the Sanscrit name is shorter and less cumbersome.

Illustrations

Plates between pages 96 and 97

Preface

In preparing this book for women our aim has been to retain the basically sane message of yoga while omitting practices unsuitable for western physique and western life. In the past, and to a certain extent even now in eastern countries, it was possible to withdraw completely from the world and dedicate the whole self to further development of body, mind and spirit; but for most westerners such an existence is out of the question. The average modern city-dweller is more likely to be living in a flat than a cave, and his way of life in varying degrees is dominated by economic circumstances.

Such people need not be excluded from the benefits of yoga, for traditional practices can be adapted without destroying their value or authenticity. Where women are concerned there are special advantages, for many of the techniques and exercises are designed to beautify face and figure and to delay old age. In this book we have concentrated on these aspects of yoga for women, though we have also dealt with the general benefits of health, strength and vitality, and the development of mental powers through simple techniques and exercises.

Due to the incessant small calls made on their attention by family and domestic life women often let their appearance go, through lack of time, lack of determination or preoccupation with things that could really be left. Some women also neglect themselves through carelessness or laziness and there is even a minority—usually middle-aged—who do it as a kind of martyrdom, as an unconscious revenge on their families or the world in general.

This sort of thing is neither necessary nor intelligent, particularly since we now have so many aids to self-improvement, mental as well as physical. Of all such aids, yoga is surely the most reliable, the safest and the best.

Women can become better-looking through yoga, not only by improving their health but through the development of a more positive interest in life and their own physical and mental problems. Most yoga teachers know cases of women who have astonished everyone, including themselves, by exchanging a drawn and harassed, middle-aged look for a youthful, vital one; by discarding stiffness and tension for suppleness, slimness, serenity and poise. In Michael Volin's yoga school in Sydney many such changes have been seen. Some changes are slow and gradual, others are quite dramatic: an actual rejuvenation in which the woman grows physically younger by years; but these cases apart, all women of any age find that yoga increases their enjoyment of life.

One of its most remarkable features is its power

to change the whole attitude to life and bring a more relaxed and serene outlook. So many women comment on the increasing calmness they feel, their ability to handle difficult situations and to give up worrying. It is a very common thing to hear pupils saying, 'I don't seem to worry any more.' This change comes about partly through mental development but also through a general improvement and toning-up of glands and relaxation of nervous centres.

For those who wish to investigate the subject in its more advanced spiritual forms there are many books of reference, but the average woman, turning to yoga as a means of improving and enriching her life, is more likely to need simple instruction, guidance and encouragement. This is what we have tried to provide. The book has been written as a collaboration and has behind it almost a quarter of a century of teaching experience. During these years Michael Volin has taught thousands of students in eastern and western countries and has had ample opportunity to observe the effects of yoga on women.

NANCY PHELAN

Sydney 1962

N.B. A certain amount of repetition has been inevitable in this book, for sometimes the same techniques or *asanas* are used for different purposes or to benefit different parts of the body. In each such case we have given the information or instructions under the relevant heading, even though it also appears elsewhere in the book, in order to help readers find information for specific purposes without having to re-read the whole book.

PART ONE

The Aims of Yoga

1

Introduction to Yoga

Yoga has often been described as a three-fold path of development, physical, mental and spiritual, for its purpose is to bring man to the highest state of advancement on all these planes. There are many different paths in yoga . . . the yoga of action, the yoga of wisdom, the yoga of knowledge, the yoga of devotion, the yoga of sounds, the yoga of higher faculties . . . but all have the same ultimate goal and all begin with hatha yoga, the philosophy of physical well-being.

This book is concerned with hatha yoga, the oldest existing physical-culture system in the world. The name *hatha* is made up of two Sanscrit roots . . . *ha*, meaning sun, and *tha*, meaning moon; and the traditional interpretation of the name is that the flow of breath through the right nostril is controlled by the sun, while that through the left is controlled by the moon. The word *yoga* means union or joining, and though it may be taken in the larger sense, referring to man's ultimate union with God or the universe, it here signifies the joining of the two breaths.

From this it will be seen that breathing is the basis

of hatha yoga. Complete control of the breath is essential to proper development and most of the movements or *asanas* (bodily positions) practised are associated with deep breathing. Mental concentration is also essential, for development of the constructive power of the mind is a vital part of training. Yogis believe that the air we breathe is transformed with a quality known as *prana* (life-force or absolute energy). This force, this extra something, which might be compared to vitamins in food, has not yet been seen or measured by scientific instruments, but it is taught that if complete control of *prana* is achieved eventually life itself may be controlled. Control of *prana* comes through control of the breath.

Apart from teaching control of the breath, the practice of yoga also brings suppleness of the spine and joints, stimulation of the glands, relaxation of the nervous centres and improvement of the digestive and eliminative powers of the body. These things are achieved through groups of *asanas*—of which there are eighty-four in number—gestures, exercises and breathing cycles. There is an exercise or *asana* for every part of the body and a student who regularly practises the greater part of them will improve in health, appearance and vitality, retaining these assets for many years. It is said that each *asana* mastered is a rebirth, and that after nine months of serious practice the body could be completely renewed.

Although hatha yoga is known as physical yoga it is not only limited to the body. Mind and spirit are equally involved. The true yogi's concern with his body is a spiritual one, for he believes that it is the temple of the living spirit and that his duty is to beautify and care for that temple to the best of his ability. Unlike the medieval religious teachers of the west who advocated mortification of the flesh, yoga believed that liberation of the spirit is more easily achieved if the body is brought to the highest state of physical perfection and under complete control of the mind.

The ultimate aim of yoga is this liberation of the spirit, the union of the soul with the universe, or soul of the universe, but in western countries only a few practise it for this purpose. The majority are content to regard it as a remarkable method of not only developing and toning-up the whole body but of delaying the process of ageing and of prolonging the creative part of life; and of developing mind and spirit by the practice of meditation and mental techniques and exercises.

There are certain yoga practices not widely known in the west which concentrate on methods of delaying old age. Some of these techniques are physical, others are mental, involving will-power, imagination and self-hypnosis, with almost a touch of magic about them. As practised in closed monasteries and *ashrams* in Tibet, India and China, they are the means by which adepts live to fantastic ages, retaining the appearance of young men. The world has always been fascinated by tales of such apparently immortal yogis and sages, of whom the greatest is Babaji, the yogi-saint, who has lived for centuries in the Himalayas, unchangingly young and beautiful.

The origin of these practices is so ancient and remote that it is surrounded in mystery. One poetic legend, told in China, tells that it was evolved by a sage at the court of a king, in order to protect his beloved from the ravages of time. So moved was he at the thought of her grace and beauty succumbing to old age that he withdrew from the world, and after sitting cross-legged, deep in trance, for three days emerged with a system designed to preserve her youth and loveliness.

Other stories suggest that they were evolved by wise men of the past, who, concerned at the brief expectation of life, set out to create a means of raising the standard of health and increasing the life-span; but the real yogi's object in prolonging the youth and strength of his body is to give his mind the longest time for development and improvement, for it is a melancholy fact that the average adult rarely begins to learn wisdom until his physical body is starting to disintegrate. Through yoga the body is, as it were, made to wait for the slower-maturing mind, so that both may reach their highest powers together, and man may enjoy a mature mind in a young and healthy body.

What yoga offers to western women

It is a remarkable fact that a system of exercises and

techniques developed thousands of years ago by eastern sages is now being practised by housewives in modern western cities. Until a few years ago these same women would have greeted the subject of yoga with blank stares, or regarded it with fear, suspicion, even ridicule. Yogis were the material for jokes and tall stories; they were unwashed, fanatical, sinister Indians who lay on beds of broken glass or sat for years with one arm up in the air. Even European yoga students were regarded with suspicion or dismissed as cranks who lived on grass and indulged in practices tinged with Black Magic.

The picture is now completely changed. In the cities and suburbs of the west women of all ages are turning to yoga, and though a certain proportion have done so because it is fashionable, the majority are serious and devoted. These women have realised that far from being a weird and dangerous oriental cult, it is a sane and natural means of improving and retaining health, appearance and enjoyment of life. The number of film-stars, artists, professional beauties and public figures of all kinds who practise yoga has brought the subject to the attention of people who otherwise might never have heard of it, but whatever the means by which she learns of it, once the average woman has encountered yoga she recognises its value.

What does this ancient physical-culture system offer to western women? How does it fit into the lives of suburban housewives, actresses and business women of all ages?

There are numerous reasons for its appeal, which vary in importance according to individual needs, but in general it might be said that it offers a means of relaxing the whole system, of beautifying and toning-up the body and of postponing the effects of old age.

All of these things have a universal appeal. Since nine out of ten adults living in western society suffer from strain, tension and maladies resulting from the exhausting demands of modern life, the ability to completely relax at will is an important asset. Since every normal woman wants to look and feel her best, to be pretty and attractive and to enjoy life to the full, a knowledge of how to achieve these things cannot fail to interest her, particularly since she knows that they can often change her whole outlook, even her life; and, finally, a means of preserving her vitality and attractions for many years is important to any woman, particularly if in the process she learns how to face old age, when it eventually comes, with serenity and charm.

How yoga works

How does yoga achieve the results claimed for it? How does it delay ageing, rejuvenate, improve appearance, maintain suppleness, increase vitality and prolong the creative part of life? Even the briefest answer to these questions reveals the fact that it is a carefully worked-out system based on a remarkable understanding of the human body and its functions.

As we have already explained, the results are achieved through control of the breath, then through a series of *asanas* and exercises which affect the whole body, the endocrine glands, the nervous system, the blood circulation, the spine, joints, muscles and internal organs. There are exercises for the mind, for the development of will-power and character, improvement of concentration and imagination. Since the exercises and *asanas* and their effects are dealt with in detail in the text of this book it will be enough to say here that women seeking to improve vitality, mental powers, sex impulses, beauty of face and figure, and retain a youthful appearance as long as possible, will find that yoga has a technique which will help in each particular problem. It does not claim to be a miracle cure-all, but rather acts as a preventive, teaching us to preserve and improve before it is too late; but in certain cases curative effects can be achieved even after damage has been done.

Age

A question very often asked is, 'What is the right age to start yoga? Am I too old?' The answer is that any age is the right age, and no one is too old, for there is a form of yoga to suit everyone. For young or middle-aged people of normal reasonable health the whole field is open; for the old or weak or ailing there are still techniques that may be safely practised, even though the most strenuous are forbidden. Everyone can practise and benefit from breathing exercises and relaxation techniques, even if high blood-pressure prevents them from standing on their heads or performing advanced raised positions; and where there are no such disabilities quite remarkable results can be achieved.

Inability to perform complicated *asanas* should not discourage students, for yoga is not competitive. It is a very individual thing and the student gets from it what she puts into it, for in this form of physical culture the mind and character are just as important as the body. A woman in her forties will often benefit far more than an immature girl, however supple, for the older woman is mentally more prepared and receptive. Physical yoga is not just a question of performing acrobatic feats and tying oneself up like a contortionist, and young people sometimes fail to realise this, thus missing the full message behind the exercises.

Sex-life and diet

There are no grounds whatever for fears that yoga will disrupt women's normal lives and turn them into anaemic ascetics. On the contrary, by toning-up the whole body it increases poise, magnetism and joy in living.

It is not necessary for anyone to become a vegetarian or a celibate unless they wish to achieve the higher forms of spiritual development and enlightenment. Women who practise yoga to improve their health, looks and general condition are only required to use common sense and moderation. (These subjects are dealt with more fully in chapters 4 and 5.)

Religion

From time to time people say they would like to practise yoga but are afraid it might conflict with their religious beliefs. This remark reveals a complete ignorance of the nature of yoga, for it does not affect anyone's religion unless to develop and intensify the capacity for religious experience and feeling. It is a philosophy, a way of life, and its whole aim is to help man reach his highest state of development. It might be described as supra-religious, in the sense that it is not tied to or limited by any one sect or faith and that its aim is universal in character. In many hatha yoga classes Protestants will be found next to Catholics, Buddhists next to Hindus, all united in following the same path towards enlightenment and development, each according to his own nature and belief.

2

The female body

It is not intended to embark on an elaborate or detailed discussion of the female body, but a brief reference to its main features and functions might help readers to understand the way in which yoga techniques and *asanas* achieve their effects.

The human body, which is made up of cells, comprises bones, muscles, tissues, nerves and organs, all enclosed and protected by the skin and to a certain extent by the skeleton, which also keeps the body upright. Within the body are various systems: the respiratory system; the digestive system; the circulatory system; the excretory system; the glandular and reproductive systems. With a remarkable knowledge and understanding of human anatomy the ancient yogis worked out methods of benefiting and developing all these systems, as well as the nervous and muscular systems, the spine and joints, the brain and mind itself.

The bony framework of the skeleton is made up of over two hundred bones, the main ones being those of the skull and face, the vertebrae of the spine, the bones of the chest and ribs, shoulders and collarbones, hip bones, arms and hands, legs and feet. The bones are connected by joints, movable and immovable and held together by cartilages and ligaments.

Certain bones have muscles attached to them, which enable them to be moved. The muscles are of two kinds—voluntary, which may be moved at will, and involuntary, which normally cannot be moved at will and which are located in the internal organs and the walls of the veins and arteries. (Advanced yogis have the ability to move and control certain involuntary muscles.) Voluntary muscles are set in pairs, a flexor and an extensor muscle, and work by contraction and relaxation of these parts. For instance, in the upper arm and biceps is the flexor muscle which contracts and raises the forearm, while the triceps is the extensor which lowers it by relaxing.

The *nervous system* and the brain have been compared to a telephone exchange where calls are received and sent. The incoming calls to the brain, registering sensations in different parts of the body, travel by the sensory nerves; the out-going calls travel by the motor nerves, carrying instructions for action to the muscles. The main line of communication between the brain and the rest of the body is the spinal cord which runs down from the head, through the backbone, protected by the vertebrae, and from which dozens of pairs of nerves branch off to the organs and other parts of the body. It will be understood from this how vital is the spinal cord, and why certain yoga *asanas* that stimulate the roots of the spinal nerves are so important.

The *respiratory system*, by which we breathe, includes the trachea or windpipe, and the lungs. Starting in the throat, the trachea branches into two bronchial tubes which lead to the lungs, where they divide up into tiny branches called alveoli, full of capillary arteries and veins. The process of breathing involves taking in oxygen needed by the body and exhaling from the lungs stale air filled with carbon dioxide discarded by the body. The oxygen enters the bloodstream from the lungs through the capillary arteries of the alveoli, and the carbon dioxide, brought to the lungs by the blood, enters them through the capillary veins and is then exhaled.

Two other essential parts of the breathing apparatus are the ribs and the diaphragm, a large flat muscle which divides the chest cavity from the abdominal region. The upwards and downwards movement of the diaphragm and the resulting expansion and contraction of the ribs creates a partial vacuum in the lungs and enables air to be drawn in through the nose, down the trachea and into the lungs. The stale air is expelled by the same action in reverse.

The *digestive system* is the mechanism by which the body is fed and nourished and consists of the alimentary canal, the liver and the pancreas. The alimentary canal includes the mouth, oesophagus, stomach, small and large intestines, all of which play a part in converting food into a form in which it can be absorbed by the cells of the body, the process known as digestion. Digestion begins in the mouth where the food, reduced to a pulpy state by the teeth, is acted on by the saliva (which digests starches). The food is then moved by the tongue into the oesophagus, through which it passes into the stomach. Here it is churned up by the muscles of the stomach walls, and, after chemical action by the digestive juices has taken place, moves into the small intestine, where it is subjected to further chemical action, including that of bile from the liver and pancreatic juice from the pancreas. Finally it is pushed into the large intestine, whence it is absorbed into the bloodstream and carried to the cells and tissues. The residue of undigested waste moves through the large intestine to the rectum and is eliminated from the body as faeces.

Heart, blood, arteries and veins are the component parts of the *circulatory system.* In its journey through the body the blood carries nourishment for the cells on the outward trip and brings back wastes and impurities on the return. The power behind this endless circuit, which ceases only with death, is the heart, which pumps the blood through the arteries to the different parts of the body and back through the veins to the heart again. The heart is a large muscle and its work of pumping the blood is done by alternating contraction and relaxation.

The blood itself contains red and white corpuscles. The red are concerned with carrying oxygen to the cells and removing carbon dioxide; the white are the body's means of fighting disease and bacteria.

The organs of the *excretory system* are the kidneys and bladder and their function is to remove liquid waste from the blood. The kidneys are in fact a fine filter system and as the blood passes through them the discarded waste it carries is separated and sent to the bladder where it is stored until passed from the body as urine.

The ductless *glands of the endocrine system* have a tremendous influence on the rest of the body, affecting not only its growth, size and shape, but also temperament, mental powers, attitude to life, energy and personality itself. The whole endocrine system is so interrelated that if one gland is out of order it can affect the balance of the rest, resulting in illness, mental or physical disorders, depression, lack of energy, loss or increase in weight. These effects are brought about by hormones which are secreted by the glands and released into the bloodstream.

The names of the endocrine glands are the pituitary, pineal, thyroid, para-thyroid, thymus, adrenals, and gonads or sex glands, which in women are represented by the ovaries. The *pituitary,* situated in the head, might be described as the controller of the glandular system, including the sex glands, and thus indirectly of the body's development, health and well-being. The *pineal* gland, also in the head but placed towards the back of the brain, helps to keep the rest of the glands in working order and in balance with one another. If, for instance, the pineal gland is destroyed the sex glands could be adversely affected. Yogis also regard the pineal gland as the seat of higher faculties, of telepathy, clairvoyance and other occult powers. The *thyroid and para-thyroid glands* are at the base of the throat and between them exert a powerful effect on the whole body, influencing vital energy, mental outlook, temperament, weight and the sex glands. Thyroid deficiency causes sluggishness, increased weight, apathy, depression, even stupidity, while over-active thyroid causes restlessness, nervousness, agitation and tension.

The *thymus gland,* lying below the thyroid and parathyroids, influences growth and development and does its work in the years before puberty. When this stage is reached it begins to shrink, otherwise normal adult development would not take place.

The hormones secreted by the *adrenal glands,* which are just above the kidneys, are responsible for vital energy, enthusiasm, drive and a positive attitude to life; while the *ovaries,* apart from their importance in the reproductive cycle, determine the powers of attraction, magnetism, confidence, warmth and feminine appeal.

In women the organs of the *reproductive system* are internal, situated in the pelvis, within the bony framework of the hips. They consist of the two ovaries, right and left, and two fallopian tubes, leading from the ovaries to the uterus, which is set in the centre and which leads into the vagina. The uterus is a small muscular organ which greatly increases in size during pregnancy and which, during childbirth, expels the child by contraction of its muscular walls.

The ovaries are two small glands situated low down on each side of the abdominal cavity, in the region of the groin, and from them come the eggs, which, fertilised by male sperm, develop into children. The eggs travel along the fallopian tubes to the uterus where, if not fertilised, they are discharged during menstruation.

In modern women these organs sometimes become disordered, causing menstrual disturbances, sexual debility, pregnancy troubles, prolapse, catarrh of the uterus and ovarian disorders; and even in the normal

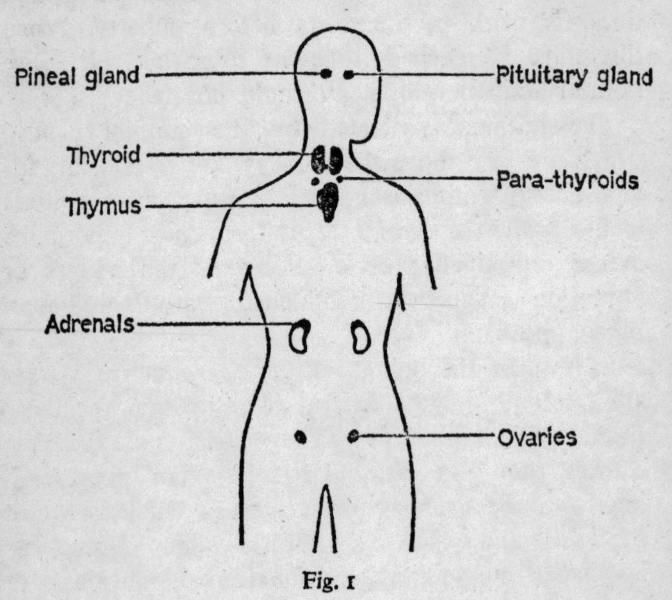

Fig. 1

course of life women often experience distressing symptoms during adolescence and change of life.

A knowledge of hatha yoga can often help these sufferers, and the table on pages 187–9 (Appendix II) will give an indication of *asanas* which are beneficial in such cases.

3

Delaying old age

From the beginning of history man has sought for a means to keep his youth. In the past alchemists searched for the Elixir of Youth, and in our own times scientists experiment to the same end with drugs and glandular extracts. From Ancient Egyptians to modern geriatricians, from Goethe to Oscar Wilde, the thought of preserving youth and beauty has obsessed mankind.

Women even more than men turn to anything that can help them delay old age . . . beauty parlours, massage, hair dyes, diets, hormone injections, cosmetic surgery, anything that can ward it off a little longer. Woman's beauty of face and form fade more quickly than man's; her skin more easily dries, her body withers. She is more susceptible to climatic hardships and often the demands of maternity help to rob her of youth.

For the average person old age cannot be held off for ever, but it can be deferred, and yoga is the only natural and efficient means we know of doing this. It must, of course, be admitted that beauty parlours are easy and a long and faithful practice of yoga is not; that beauty parlours require no effort on your part and yoga demands full concentration and application; that in the beauty parlour you can lie back without a care, while in yoga, especially in the mental exercises, you must work hard; but the difference in results cannot be compared. Artificial means are only temporary second-best. Beauty parlours cannot really make the blood flow back into withered tissues, or permanently firm up sagging muscles, whereas yoga can and does. We have already spoken of the legendary yogis of the east who preserve a youthful appearance up to fantastic ages, and even outside the *ashrams* and closed monasteries there are many extraordinary cases of this victory over time. One of Michael Volin's teachers in China, a Tibetan-Chinese yogi named Hoo Pei who was famous for his knowledge of breathing, when over seventy looked no more than forty; and a recent example, closer to home, is the case of a woman doctor living in London, who, by mastering certain advanced techniques involving self-hypnosis, preserved a young and beautiful appearance well into her fifties.

The average European woman would not have the time or will-power to master these mysterious techniques, nor does she aspire to live for centuries. She is quite satisfied if she can retain a good proportion of her youth and looks to the end of her life. For her the best to be had is a slowing down of the process, a postponing of the time when she must succumb to old age, but when this time does come she can, with the help of yoga, turn it into victory instead of defeat by ageing gracefully and gently. An autumn flower can be just as lovely as a spring flower; and autumnnal beauty even more moving than the firm freshness of youth; and a woman whose physical body has aged gradually, yet whose spirit has grown clearer and stronger with time, has an incandescent quality unknown to her in youth. Like an alabaster vase lit from within, her face is illuminated by the beauty of wisdom, experience and understanding.

Even if women cannot devote their whole time to fighting old age, there are many who would emulate an elderly woman in a Sydney class, who, starting yoga in her seventies, on medical advice, became fifteen years younger, biologically, in less than a year, according to the testimony of her astonished doctor.

Apart from such cases of actual rejuvenation, the practice of yoga is said to slow down ageing considerably. This slowing down is the basis for the yogi's belief that the springtime of man's life is from fifty-five to seventy-five; a statement supported in our own day by geriatricians, who claim that with the help of scientific discoveries Wimbledon tennis finals of the future will be played by people in their sixties.

Yoga achieves its slowing-down effects by considering every aspect of ageing in the human body and using different means to check them. It fights against central gravity forces which all through life exert a downward pull on the body, causing tissues to sag and internal organs to become displaced, particularly in women; it can delay the menopause, and through its effect on the glands has even been known to restore menstruation in ageing women; it feeds facial tissues and skin, which, starved of blood by poor circulation, become lined and wrinkled; it refreshes the nervous system by the practice of relaxation; it recharges the body and purifies the bloodstream by breathing exercises; it preserves the vital energy by improving the quality of sleep; and finally it holds off old age by the power of the mind, the greatest and most subtle power in the body.

There is nothing mysterious in these physical techniques; you are simply taking each part of the body in turn and repairing the damage done to it by time, abuse, lack of care, over-strain. It is not necessary to accept premature physical destruction as permanent; things can be repaired by proper treatment. When, for example, we consider men who, prematurely aged during the war by frightful hardship, regained youth, strength and physical beauty by rest, correct diet and sunshine, we find it easier to accept yoga's teaching that anyone can prolong the best part of life as long as he wishes.

Let us first consider the physical methods of delaying old age.

The pull of *central gravity,* with its resultant ageing effects, is counteracted by the practice of inverted positions. These include the Shoulderstand, Half-shoulderstand and the Headstands (pages 131, 133 and 135). Sagging muscles, prolapses, varicose veins, are all discouraged and improved by these *asanas*, provided, of course, there is no physical disability, such as high blood-pressure, to forbid practising them.

Facial tissues and the skin of the face are the first things to show signs of ageing, for as we get older the blood does not circulate so freely in these areas as it does in youth. The result is a drawn, pale and wrinkled appearance. When you compare the glowing skin and firm fresh face of a healthy child with that of an old person, thin and white like paper, you will understand how important it is for these facial tissues to receive adequate nourishment from the bloodstream if they are to remain firm and unlined.

Regular practise of the Headstand and, above all, of the Half-shoulderstand will help to prevent and destroy wrinkles. In the Half-shoulderstand the blood drained from the upraised legs flows to the face, suffusing it and feeding the starving tissues.

Other *asanas* which have the effect of bringing blood to the face and head are: Yoga-*mudra* (page 154); Pose of a Child (page 154); Head of a Cow (page 153); Bird Pose (page 146) and Pose of a Raven (page 147); Head-to-knee pose—standing and sitting (page 139); the stretching cycle (page 137), and various breathing exercises, including the *Ha* or Cleansing Breath. There are also several simple, preliminary techniques, such as swinging forward and downwards from the waist, which brings extra blood to the face, and an exercise in which the head is flushed with blood. This is practised lying on the back. Inhale, bring the knees to the stomach and press them close to the body with the hands, holding the pose until you feel the blood going to the face. Then exhale and lower legs. (This is also recommended for flatulence.)

The glands affecting the sex functions are kept young and healthy by the inverted poses, and by other *asanas* which tone-up the reproductive system (see Chapter 4). Of these the most important are the Shoulderstand and the Headstand, which practised sufficiently can delay the menopause and prolong creative sex-life.

Relaxation

Mastery of relaxation technique for completely resting muscles, nerves and mind is essential in retaining a youthful appearance. No woman can hope to keep her looks or youth if she wears a tense or harassed expression; if to the lines caused by starved tissues are added lines of strain round eyes and mouth, and an unattractive hardness and brittleness. Practise *Savasana* (Pose of Complete Rest) as described on page 119 as often as you can if you wish to avoid these things. Correct relaxation is just as beneficial as sleep. A most important factor in delaying old age is the gradual accumulation of life energy or vitality, increasing your supply rather than letting it decrease, which is the case with many people. This is not hard to do; it is just a matter of getting enough sleep, exercise and fresh air. Most adults live under a constant weight of accumulated tiredness, caused by restless sleep, late nights, unventilated rooms, unwise diet or too much smoking and drinking.

Make an effort to get rid of this undischarged tiredness and these impurities. Make up your mind to have at least two early nights, going to bed when the children go; try to break the habit of staying up too late, to read or sew or watch television, insidious things, which, harmless in themselves, can ruin your total of sleeping hours.

Remember that your body contains many muscles, which must be exercised. Watch your diet. Try to have fruit-juice days or fasting days (see Chapter 5) to purify the system, but be careful not to overdo them. Women who are no longer young can make themselves look older instead of younger if they lose too much weight too suddenly.

Do not let yourself become constipated, for impurities collected in the bloodstream, through incomplete elimination, will destroy your health, vitality and looks. Researchers specialising in geriatrics are now of the opinion that such incomplete elimination is one of the main causes of ageing, for the poisons left in the body are re-absorbed through the walls of the bowels into the blood, with destructive effect on the tissues. In this, modern scientists and ancient yogis are in complete agreement, for one of the most important of yoga teachings is that the body must be kept internally clean and free of impurities if it is to stay young.

Avoid heavy and starchy foods, if your eliminative system is sluggish, and practise the *asanas* listed on page 82 for constipation.

These things will help you preserve, even increase, your vital energy, apart from the toning-up effects of the *asanas* on the organs and nerves of the body; and it is this vital energy which will keep you young. Direct it into constructive channels . . . be always occupied, interested, alert, optimistic. To be occupied does not mean running about in the physical sense but to be always positive in your reaction to life. Even relaxation can be practised in a positive or a negative way and the results entirely depend on which way you choose to do it.

Mental techniques in delaying old age

Even if a woman works to preserve her appearance, practising the physical methods we have described, she will not fully succeed in attaining her objective unless she can keep her mind and personality young.

Middle-age often descends upon women halfway through their thirties; they give up, sink into inertia, lose interest and become unhappy, unsatisfied and neurotic. Often by the time her children are old enough to appreciate her as a person a mother has become a dull and pathetic old woman, full of grudges and ailments to which she clings by way of compensation for her lost charms. Doctors' surgeries and psychoanalysts' rooms are full of such women, and those who cannot afford this kind of solace often vent their bitterness and disappointment on the wives of their sons, jealous of their youth.

This is an everyday occurrence and the sad thing is that it need not happen. A woman who looks after herself sensibly, not only preserving her vitality and interest in her appearance but also retaining a fresh and positive attitude to life, never sinks into this condition. It is not necessary to be rich or even to lead a life of leisure; the main requirements are patience, determination and perseverance; but there are still many women who cannot accept these simple truths, who will not try, who hang back, miserable and discontented, spoiling the lives of their families as well as their own.

There is no excuse for this sort of thing, particularly now when the general attitude to age is so different from that of the past. At one time forty was considered old. Shakespeare wrote:

> 'When forty winters shall beseige thy brow,
> And dig deep trenches in thy beauty's field . . .'

and earlier Xenophon described how, on the return from the Persian expedition, he secured ships for the women, the sick and *those over forty*. No adult now really believes he is old at forty, and by yoga standards it is barely the springtime of life. (Yoga teaches that the physical body is still developing until the age of thirty-three.)

We have said that the advanced mental techniques used in delaying old age are far beyond the average woman's capabilities, but there is nothing to prevent anyone doing the more elementary exercises, provided there is confidence in their power to help. This should not be hard to achieve. Every woman knows that at certain times of her life her appearance varies . . . that she looks younger or older according to stimulus or boredom; that happiness and interest are rejuvenating and depression and monotony are ageing. If happiness and depression—which, after all, are states of mind—can make us appear younger or older without any conscious effort on our part, what is so strange about a really concentrated mental attitude affecting our appearance? When the vitality is low we look tired, feel colourless and convey this impression to those we meet; when vitality is high we communicate it to others in dynamic power and personal magnetism. We can influence other people to our way of thinking purely by personality if we have sufficient self-confidence; we can destroy our advantages by a gloomy and pessimistic attitude.

The first thing to do is to develop the right general attitude to the subject, concentrating on the thought, 'I will not let myself get older,' never saying, as so many people do, 'I am getting old,' even to yourself. This is not done as a wild defiance of something inevitable, but as a slowing down method, a general discouragement to the encroachment of old age.

The next thing is to give up worrying, and though this may sound an unreal suggestion it can be made an actual fact. Mental techniques and the development of a more philosophical attitude to life (see mental exercises in Chaper 6) are more than half the battle against worrying, but it is astonishing how much help your own body can give if you allow it. As we mentioned at the beginning of this book, one of the most noticeable effects of yoga is its power to change one's whole attitude to life, and over and over again people—particularly women—have suddenly discovered that after some months of practice they are no longer worrying about things as they did before. It almost seems as though the apparatus used for this entirely negative and destructive occupation has been dulled or destroyed, but the truth is that proper exercise and regular toning-up of glands and nerves have stimulated and relaxed the body and mind, resulting in a far more serene attitude to life.

There are several simple but effective mental exercises which will help you to slow down ageing if you give them a chance, and they should be supplemented by those in the section on mental hygiene (pages 101–4). Though at first glance they may not all appear connected with rejuvenation you will find that they are so in a subtle and slightly more indirect way than physical techniques. All should be practised sitting in a comfortable cross-legged position, with steady and rhythmical breath established as described on pages 122–33.

1. *Mind mirror*

Concentrate all your thoughts upon seeing before you

the image of yourself, as you are now, as clearly as though looking in a mirror. Then project this image into the future, unchanged, unchangeable through the years to come. Every detail of your present appearance should be vividly seen in the mind's eye, and kept as it is now, in your projection into the future. This exercise, and the one that follows, are simple forms of self-hypnosis, an elementary stage in the techniques we have mentioned that are used by advanced yogis to prolong youth and beauty for fantastic periods.

2. In the second part of this exercise you commence by seeing yourself in the mind mirror, as above, but then instead of projecting into the future, you see yourself the same but younger, as you were ten, fifteen, twenty years before. Holding the younger image firmly in the mind's eye, try to fit it over your present image, sliding them together so that they completely merge, as though bringing something sharply into focus, and until the younger image has quite replaced the present one.

3. *Concentration on beauty*

Yoga teaches that beauty is everywhere if one can learn to see it, and that complete concentration upon a beautiful thought, scene or object will result in relaxation of the mind and achievement of tranquillity.

In this exercise try to picture a beautiful landscape, entirely detached from your normal life, and concentrate your whole mind upon it, not in the way of trying to note details or features but rather of sheer enjoyment and appreciation of its peace and loveliness. The effect of this exercise might be compared to suddenly arriving in a serene and sheltered place after a rough and terrible journey.

4. In the second part of this exercise try to actually see yourself in this lovely place, free of care and responsibility, completely happy. Yoga believes that in doing this one relaxes the subconscious mind by escaping from the usual environment.

5. *Concentration on the object of love and devotion*
The subject of this meditation can be widely interpreted, according to the practitioner's personal life and temperament. She concentrates her whole thought upon the object she loves the most, and whether it is child, husband, parent, friend, an ideal, an object of religious devotion, God Himself, does not matter, for it is the feeling of love evoked that is important, not its cause. Pure and selfless love is the greatest illuminator of all and this inner radiance lights up and transforms the most commonplace features with a luminous beauty.

6. *Attunement to universal goodness*
Everyone has a moment in which they feel so at one with themselves and all life that their only desire is to be good, to hurt no one, to love everyone and

everything. This blessed state was known to many saints but for most of us it is a fleeting and infrequent experience. Through yoga we can learn to reach this consciousness of universal goodness at will. As you sit concentrating, try to turn all your mental powers upon the thought of universal goodness of everything that stands for goodness in your mind, and then, as though tuning in to some mysterious broadcast, try to feel yourself sharing in it, absorbing it, becoming part of it.

7. *Directing* prana *to different parts of the body*
Evoke the image of yourself, as described in mind mirror, and carefully consider each feature, each part of the body, critically appraising them. Having decided which needs help or rejuvenation, direct *prana* to that part, sending it, as you exhale, to face or thighs or any limb you choose. As you direct the *prana* in this way concentrate upon the thought that the selected part is actually improving, growing firmer, younger, clearer. . . . You can take each part needing attention and concentrate upon it in turn—for instance crows' feet round the eyes or lines on the forehead—and devote a period to its rejuvenation and improvement.

8. *Sending a goodwill message to the vital organs*
As we know, the body is made up of cells. Yoga teaches that each of these cells has an instinctive mind which can be trained to respond to the master mind in

the brain. The yogi's knowledge and control of these instinctive minds is one of his means of preserving his body. Having established your steady pose and rhythmical breathing, concentrate upon sending from your master mind messages and instructions to the instinctive minds in your vital organs . . . to stomach, liver, kidneys or whichever part may be working sluggishly or ineffectively. In this way try to improve digestion, discourage constipation, help a tired heart or weak lungs.

There are several very ancient exercises for increasing vital energy, drawing *prana* from the earth, from the air and from water, and transferring it to your own body; also of absorbing vital force from the sun.

1. Sit under a tree, in some secluded place, cross-legged and with hands resting on the knees. The thumb and index finger are closed (see pictures of cross-legged poses) and the other fingers are stretched out straight to make contact with the earth. Inhale, absorbing strength from the earth; exhale, transferring it to yourself.

2. Sitting cross-legged, with arms held up above the head and parallel to each other, inhale, concentrating on drawing energy from the ether, through the finger-tips; exhale, transferring it to your own store of vitality.

3. Floating in the water, breathing rhythmically; inhale, absorbing energy through the pores of the body. As you exhale, transfer it to yourself.

4. Energy from the sun. This is best done in the early morning, when the sun is not very strong. Sit exposed to the sun wearing as few clothes as possible. Turn the body 90 degrees every five, ten or fifteen minutes, according to the strength of the sun, so that in twenty minutes you have completed a circle, exposing the whole body to the sun. Inhale, absorbing its energy; exhale, transferring it to yourself.

4

Yoga and sex

A woman's body plays a far more complex part in her life than a man's does in his. However advanced she may become spiritually, her body continues to make its demands on her attention; it goes through a series of processes that she cannot ignore—puberty, menstruation, menopause and usually pregnancy and childbirth; it develops maladies unknown to male bodies; it ages more quickly than a man's and it exerts an undeniable influence upon her whole character. A woman who feels herself physically unattractive is usually diffident, inhibited and full of complexes, in contrast to a pretty woman who is sure of herself and her power to attract.

In nature's plan a woman's primary function is to produce children. No matter how much talent, brains, artistic genius she may also possess her chief physical purpose is to continue the race and to this end she must find a mate. The drive towards mating, which is healthy and natural, is the instinct behind a normal woman's wish to look attractive, whether she realises it or not.

Contrary to popular opinion, yoga does not forbid or discourage sex. Many people believe that the practice of yoga will either oblige them to give up a normal sex-life or will destroy their sex impulses; they are surprised to hear that many great yogis of the past have been house-holders and family men, and that certain *asanas* and practices are recommended for the improvement and greater enjoyment of sex.

Those who wish to follow the highest forms of spiritual yoga, to submit themselves to the discipline of an *ashram* or heritage, must indeed lead a celibate life, but this is not for any moralistic reason nor does it mean that the sex impulse is repressed. Yogis have discovered that sex energy, conserved and sublimated, increases mental and psychic powers, and they have devised techniques of sublimation whereby normal sex impulses are transmuted into mental and psychic energy. This is the reason for a celibate life; but the ordinary western student who is not seeking to develop these mysterious faculties is not expected to follow such practices. On the contrary, such students find that yoga benefits their sex-life by teaching relaxation, increasing vitality and toning-up the sex glands. Where women are concerned it can also help them in a therapeutic way, certain *asanas* having a powerful effect on the female reproductive system and thereby correcting disorders and abnormalities in these organs.

As far as the female physical part of their lives is concerned, most healthy women have very little difficulty, but there are others who suffer endlessly. They have trouble in adolescence, painful menstruation all through maturity, difficult or unsuccessful pregnancies and miserable change of life. Often there are definite physical reasons for this suffering, but in many cases it could be cured or alleviated by a sensible and positive attitude. We are concerned here with the physical remedies which will bring relief—the mental aspects are dealt with more fully in Chapter 6—but it must be emphasised that in yoga, mind and body must work together if there are to be complete results. No amount of exercises will really succeed if the constructive power of the mind is not employed at the same time.

Adolescence

Many young girls entering into physical maturity have trouble with menstruation. Sometimes the periods do not appear, sometimes they start and then vanish and at other times they are painful and profuse. Menstrual troubles are not the only trials of adolescence; girls become over-weight, their complexions become blotchy and often disfigured with pimples and acne; their movements are gauche and clumsy, they feel restless, awkward, unhappy; they are full of vague disturbing instincts and develop all kinds of complexes, mainly inferiority. They are no longer children, glad of parental protection, yet they are not adults, free to do as they like. They mope and become melancholy or they hate and defy everyone. They believe themselves martyred and misunderstood and sometimes drift into serious trouble as a result.

A doctor should always be consulted about menstrual irregularities, but provided there is no physical reason to forbid it, yoga can also help the growing girl. Not only do some of the *asanas* have beneficial effects on menstruation through the glands, but practice in general will improve the whole bodily condition, relaxing the nerves and thus helping reduce the miseries of adolescence, and by improving the appearance, regulating the weight and clearing the complexion, will give the young girl a feeling of poise and confidence she would otherwise lack.

This psychological change, due to improvement of the physical condition, is a common occurrence, and an example was noticed while this book was being written. In a class of slim and pretty girls there was one pupil who was fat, clumsy and plain. She spoke to no one, sat at the back of the room and could never be persuaded to try any *asana,* such as the Headstand, if the other girls could see her. She was surly and reserved and always left the room as soon as the class was over.

After five or six weeks she suddenly began to change. Her weight decreased noticeably, and when the other girls remarked on it in a friendly way she did not scowl in her former manner but smiled and thanked them pleasantly. The next week she came wearing lipstick for the first time and a week later she had her hair cut and set in a becoming way. She began to look quite pretty, and as her figure improved, her dressing, which had been dowdy and negative, also improved. Not only was her appearance affected but her confidence increased and one day she surprised the class by volunteering to do the Headstand, executing it so well that it was clear she had been practising at home. Her response to the other girls' congratulations was natural and relaxed, showing that her attitude to them and to life in general had completely changed. Twelve weeks after starting yoga lessons she was almost transformed and it is obvious that she is now a much happier girl.

The most important postures for correcting menstrual and adolescent troubles are Shoulderstand (page 131); Fish (page 143); Plough (page 139); Cobra (page 142); Locust (page 143); Half-shoulderstand (page 133); Supine Pelvic (page 145); Headstand (page 135); Head-to-knee Pose, standing and sitting (page 139), and *Savasana* or Position of Complete Rest (page 117). Instructions for performing them are given on the pages shown above.

Pregnancy (see also Appendix I. Yoga and natural childbirth).

Apart from exercises specifically practised for the purpose of facilitating natural childbirth, normal women in the earlier stages of pregnancy can benefit from yoga, keeping supple, healthy and cheerful in the process. Such things as pictures of a well-known film-star performing the Shoulderstand in the seventh month of pregnancy, under the direction of her doctor-husband, have helped to dispel many women's doubts about the safety of taking such exercise, though everyone may not be able to carry it to such lengths. With a doctor's approval, relaxation, breathing cycles, some of the forward-stretching and inverted poses and all the cross-legged positions could be practised.

Expectant mothers are advised to use their discretion and common sense in exercising, to avoid anything that involves strenuous upward-stretching, not to practise the stomach contractions, *Uddiyana* and *Nauli,* and after the first few months to give up standing on the head, lest the child be displaced. For the rest they may continue to exercise as long as they comfortably can, with special emphasis on breathing and relaxation.

Menopause

Sooner or later every woman must go through the menopause or change of life, when her period of childbearing and menstruation come to an end. In the past, when sex was shrouded in mystery and mentioned only in whispers, there were many confused and ignorant ideas about this natural process, some women even believing it involved complete loss of femininity and the development of such masculine characteristics as a beard and a deep voice. Even now, when these subjects are treated so much more frankly and sanely, there are still women who enter upon the menopause believing they are entering into hell.

Often this is just what they are doing, but it is largely

a self-made hell, brought about by their own state of mind; for although the process is a physical one, many of its symptoms and sufferings are psychological. Once this fact has been accepted an intelligent woman has a weapon for helping her in the fight against an inevitable and sometimes merciless enemy.

There is no definite rule about the age at which change of life begins, but it is generally between forty-five and fifty-five, though it has been known to start much earlier. It is said that the longer a woman continues to bear children the later will the menopause begin. Whatever the age, the physical process is the same. The ovaries cease to produce the egg-cells, which, fertilised by the male sperms, grow into children; menstruation comes to an end, sometimes suddenly, sometimes gradually. Often there are hot flushes, giddiness, palpitation, insomnia, depression and unreasonable irritability . . . symptoms which vary in different women. If to these physical disturbances are added psychological fears and anxieties the result is often extreme suffering, sometimes causing complete lack of balance and even insanity. Even in mild cases women can become temporarily deranged, giving themselves over to jealousy, envy, hatred and self-pity. They become wrought up to such a state of tension that they can no longer control themselves and indulge in frenzied rages that are exhausting and humiliating. They are, at these times, not really responsible for their actions, but though this much may be conceded, it is their responsibility to try to prevent themselves reaching the stage where such strong emotions overwhelm them. In many cases, where women have lived a full and busy life, these disagreeable symptoms are negligible but spoilt and indolent women who have too much time and too little occupation often become an easy prey to them.

This difficult period of life, whether it comes naturally or through surgery, can be improved by a determination to overcome it to the best of one's ability. Medically there are the use of sedatives and hormone treatment, but some doctors now regard hormone injections with distrust, claiming that they encourage internal growths. The only completely safe way of improving the condition is the practice of yoga.

Yoga will not give overnight results, nor will its benefits be achieved easily, but regular practice will bring much relief. In many cases the *asanas* have actually delayed the menopause by stimulating the sex glands, and in others they have even been known to restore menstruation after it had stopped. No woman really wants to lose her sex attractions, and if it is possible to postpone this fate she feels justified in doing so; on the other hand, refusal to accept the inevitable will result in misery, and it is only by developing a calm and philosophical attitude towards this stage of life that women can successfully weather it. It is in achieving this tranquil state of mind that yoga can help.

Daily practice of *Savasana* (relaxation) and deep breathing will help to combat insomnia and nervous anxiety, and to reduce the tension that so often finds expression in emotional outbursts. Mental techniques combined with deep breathing will help to develop a more philosophical outlook and practice of the *asanas*, apart from those directly affecting the sex organs, will generally tone up the body so that inescapable symptoms give the minimum of discomfort.

As well as these measures, women could lessen some of their menopausal miseries by the use of common sense. If the system is upset and unbalanced, resulting in tensions, it stands to reason that extra stimulants will exaggerate the trouble. Alcohol is not good at this time, for it not only stimulates the body and thus increases its unpleasant symptoms, but it destroys self-control and causes people to say and do things they often regret. Many scenes and quarrels might never occur at all if it were not for alcohol taken at the wrong time, and when a woman is already fighting an unnatural tendency towards such things, as she often is during change of life, she is helping to destroy herself if she does anything to facilitate their occurrence. Some people even go so far as to forbid tea and coffee, and though this seems rather extreme in most cases it is certainly advisable not to take them at night if you find them stimulating, or at any time if they cause indigestion or over-heating of the blood.

You should try to find time to rest and relax each day. It is not always easy to do so, but it can be done, as so many busy people have proved. Keep yourself occupied and your mind alert; if your children no longer need you fill your life with hobbies; with gardening, reading, exercising, with trying to help other people, as individuals or through charitable organisations. Do not lose interest in your appearance, your grooming, your clothes. Fight to preserve your balance, your optimism and, above all, your sense of humour, for this last is perhaps your most vital weapon against all your ills.

Practise *Savasana* several times a day (page 117); deep breathing cycles (page 124); mental exercises (pages 48–52); Shoulderstand (page 131); and Half-shoulderstand (page 133); will help to counteract hot flushes and so will the Plough (page 139), the cross-legged poses (pages 128–30) and the Headstand (page 135), providing there is no indication of high blood-pressure. (Women going through the menopause should have their blood-pressure checked regularly and if it is above normal practice of *Savasana* will help to reduce it.)

Menstrual disorders

Menstrual troubles are not confined to adolescents; many adult women suffer from painful or irregular periods all their lives. In these cases, after medical approval has been given, the condition can be improved by the practice of certain *asana*, listed below. It must be pointed out, however, that to get fullest benefits the sufferer should not limit herself to these positions only but follow the general pattern of practice, for the other exercises will tone up her whole body and generally raise her state of health, mental and physical. She should also take plenty of rest, and regular vaginal douches made up of warm salted water (one teaspoon of salt to one pint of warm water). This solution is harmless and beneficial.

The *asanas* recommended for menstrual troubles are: Bow (page 142); Cobra (page 142); Shoulder-stand (page 131); Fish (page 143); Plough (page 139); Locust (page 143); Head-to-knee Pose (page 139) and stomach contractions (page 147). Relaxation and breathing cycles should also be included.

Sexual debility

Sexual debility should not be confused with frigidity, which is usually psychological in origin. The former is more a loss of sexual drive, a weakening of impulses and general lack of interest in sex. Some women do not care if this happens: they are glad to direct their energies into other channels and live a peaceful, almost celibate, existence, but there are others who are distressed by the condition, fearing it will affect their marriages. These fears can cause neuroses, anxiety, headaches, bad temper and even nervous breakdowns, and apart from robbing women of a normal part of life, usually cause domestic unhappiness and friction. It is always advisable to see a doctor in such cases, for there is the possibility of physical causes (anaemia, for instance); but if there is no serious medical reason for the trouble it will improve with proper diet, rest, relaxation and the practice of breathing exercises. The *asanas* recommended are Shoulderstand (page 131); Half-shoulderstand (page 133); Headstand (page 135); Plough (page 139); Fish (page 143); Supine Pelvic (page 145); also stomach contractions (page 147); *Aswini-mudra* (page 154) and *Yoga-mudra* (page 154); Spinal Twist (page 141).

A more subtle exercise, involving re-direction of *prana* in the body, is to lie down flat on the floor, completely relaxed, placing fingertips lightly on the region of the solar plexus. Establish deep and rhythmical breathing and form a mental image of *prana* being drawn in with inhalation and directed with exhalation through the fingertips into the solar plexus. Imagine you are literally recharging the battery of the body, increasing the amount of life-force. (This exercise is based on the belief that as we are normally inhaling and exhaling the amount of *prana* is circulating through the nervous channels, but part of it escapes into the atmosphere through the fingertips. When they are on the solar plexus the circuit of *prana* is closed in the body, and instead of escaping it is returned to the seat of vitality.)

After holding this position for several minutes place the hands alongside the body and continuing your deep and rhythmical breathing think that with *inhalation* you are drawing extra accumulated life-force from the solar plexus, and with exhalation you are directing it to the region of the reproductive organs.

Sterility

The practice of yoga has so often had beneficial effects on sterile couples that women sometimes say facetiously that they fear to take it up lest they become pregnant.

The poses listed for sexual debility and menstrual troubles should be practised, the inverted group for their power to stimulate the sex glands through the thyroid or pituitary, and the rest for their direct effect on the ovaries. An additional *asana* recommended is Eagle Pose (page 152), in which the position of the body and legs puts pressure on these glands.

Apart from actual stimulation of the reproductive system the whole body will be strengthened and health benefited so that conditions for pregnancy become more favourable. There are many cases in which women who have had a series of miscarriages through constitutional weaknesses have so improved that pregnancy no longer becomes a strain.

Sex-life

It will be clear from this chapter that the practice of yoga can help the attainment and enjoyment of a normal and healthy sex-life, directly as well as indirectly. Many women do not seem to realise how important their general state of health is in these matters; they allow themselves to become anaemic, exhausted and nervy through bad diet or lack of rest and then cannot understand why they no longer have an interest in sex; others develop complexes and inhibitions which either destroy their pleasure in life or turn them into sexual cripples.

In this age of psycho-analysis and free talk about sex it should not be necessary to remind women that it is a natural part of life and no more to be hidden than eating or sleeping, but unfortunately there are still many who retain an unreal attitude to the subject. It is from these unhappy women that harsh and bigoted attitudes to sex have come, not from ascetic yogis, who though refraining from sex themselves do not condemn it in others.

On the other hand too much interest is as bad as none, and there is nothing so trying as the kind of woman with a morbid interest in her own and everyone else's reproductive organs, and whose whole conversation is conducted in furtive whispers and suggestive references.

Yoga's main injunction in sex, as in everything, is to practise moderation, to avoid excess; to have the right mental attitude . . . positive, open, free of guilty feelings; to observe physical and mental cleanliness, and to improve the general quality of sex by raising the tone of the whole body, as well as stimulating deficient sex glands.

To enjoy your sex-life to the full you need good health and vitality, and to keep these things you should give them a little time and thought. There are many people who get along quite well without taking any care of themselves, sometimes, in exceptional cases, they retain their health and vigour until they die; but usually such people are worn out by middle-age. With a little sense anyone can avoid this fate and enjoy life for many years.

To keep well, strong and happy, follow a sensible diet, take adequate rest and adequate exercise. Attend to your appearance, your face and figure, your clothes and grooming. Keep your mind alert and interested and your outlook tolerant and optimistic. Such *asanas* as the inverted cycle, including the Headstand, and others listed in this chapter will increase your sexual vitality and keep your sex glands healthy.

A happy sex-life can be destroyed by worry, tension, nervous conditions, lack of confidence and the emotional states resulting from these things. The regular practice of *Savasana* and deep-breathing cycles, of Triangular Pose (page 133) and if possible the Lotus Position (page 129) will help to improve these conditions, and mental exercises for developing inner strength and serenity (pages 48–52 and 100–4) will discourage jealousy, possessiveness and other destructive emotions. Mental control is the hardest of all to achieve, much harder than any physical *asanas* or exercises, but if it can be attained it will bring such remarkable changes into your life that you will never regret the work you put into it.

Internal hygiene

Many women who keep the outside of their bodies clean and well exercised consider any mention of internal female hygiene indecent and repulsive, regarding a vaginal douche as sinful and appalled at the thought of vaginal exercises. In some minds internal hygiene is vaguely linked with thoughts of self-gratification, in others it just inspires revulsion, and this kind of ignorance and prejudice inhibits a healthy attitude to the subject, which, after all, is no more sinful than cleaning the teeth or washing the face.

Vaginal douches of warm water, or warm water with a little salt, should be part of every woman's toilet, not reserved for illness or for contraceptive purposes. They should not be overdone, should not be taken too hot or too cold or with strong antiseptic solutions in them. Salt and water is better than soap and water, though a weak solution with an olive-oil soap will not do any harm. If you do not know how to take a douche you should ask a doctor or nurse to show you, though most women have no difficulty in managing it, and you should use for preference the type of douche in which the water runs down from a can or hot-water bottle, rather than a syringe type, which is not so clean or effective. If you live in a country where *bidets* are part of the normal bathroom furniture your task will be made much easier.

Do not be influenced by women who tell you that douching is dangerous or unnatural. It is not dangerous if done properly and if strong disinfectants are not used, and as far as the second claim is concerned it is a matter of one unnatural practice counteracting another. It is not really natural for us to wear clothes, and if women's sex organs were exposed to the sun and air there would be less necessity for baths, douches, scents and soaps.

In addition to *asanas* for toning up the sex glands —given in this chapter—there is a technique which, intended for both sexes, can be adapted by women for their own physiology. In this exercise, known as *Aswini-mudra* (page 154), which is combined with deep breathing, the muscles of the anus are contracted and relaxed alternately, gradually reaching a strong and elastic condition where a number of contractions may be practised successively. In women the muscles at the front of the rectum lie next to those in the back wall of the vagina, and having become accustomed to *Aswini-mudra,* women can learn to concentrate on contraction and relaxation of the vagina itself, in the same way, thus keeping it firm and elastic and repairing any stretching done in childbirth. As well as toning-up the vaginal muscles these contractions are very beneficial when used in intercourse.

Sublimation

For those who cannot lead a normal sex-life there are two alternatives: repression or sublimation. Repression is bad, often resulting in all kinds of illnesses, mental and physical, in warped personalities and, in extreme cases, in vicious crimes. Sublimation, on the other hand, can only be beneficial, for it is nothing more than the transmuting of one form of energy into another; a means of direction into constructive channels a vitality which, if depressed, could become destructive.

Advanced yogis have many techniques for achieving sublimation and a very austere and rigid way of life is imposed upon disciples in *ashrams* and monasteries. As we have explained, this is not done to mortify the flesh but to conserve all vital energy, including sex energy, for transmuting into mental and psychic powers. Even erotic dreams are prohibited for the possible loss of semen they might occasion.

Yoga students living in western society are not concerned with these techniques, but there is a simple exercise in sublimation which if practised seriously will help an unhappy, unfulfilled woman to attain peace of mind. The most suitable time to practise it is when she is most disturbed by sex impulses which she cannot satisfy, but it can also be done at other times. It requires considerable will-power and determination, but the practitioner will have positive results if she can believe that it is not just a soothing and meaningless formula but will really help her on the physical plane.

Sit in a cross-legged position, the Lotus if you can manage it in comfort, with back and neck in one straight line. Establish deep and rhythmical breathing for a few minutes: then concentrate all your mind and will-power on sublimation. As you inhale, believe that you are literally drawing the energy from your sex organs, and, as you exhale, directing it to the solar plexus, which is the seat of vital energy in the human body. What you are doing is taking the energy from a centre where it is causing disturbance because it cannot find an outlet, and moving it to another centre from which it can be expressed as increased vitality, magnetism and power. The same energy can be directed similarly to the brain, resulting in greater mental powers. (This is the reverse of the exercise given on pages 64–5, for sexual debility.)

If you feel the need for sublimation do not brush aside this simple technique as nonsense. Try it, seriously and continuously, and see what happens.

Other ways of helping with this problem are to occupy the mind, keep yourself busy and avoid things that stimulate sex instincts . . . alcohol, rich foods, prolonged hot baths. Keep in the open air as much as possible, take plenty of exercise and, if you can, direct your energies into some active sport, which is a healthy, harmless and efficient form of sublimation. Finally, try to find an objective in your life that will fill your attention and give you an absorbing goal to aim at.

5

Diet

Women who have been practising hatha yoga for some time often look with surprise at books, articles and advertisements for freak diets, slimming pills, reducing machines, hot-boxes and so on. They realise that there is no need for these extreme measures if excess weight is taken in time, or, better still, never allowed to accumulate. If women could prevent themselves getting too fat in youth they would escape much unhappiness, for once the skin has been stretched for years to accommodate large quantities of fat it never regains its elasticity, and when the weight is lost it becomes flaccid, wrinkled and loose. Even for those who are not abnormally fat, exercise is essential during reducing diets if the body is to remain reasonably firm. There is nothing so ugly as the upper arms of a woman who has lost weight and never exercised; the skin hangs like an empty sack when the arm is lifted and falls into wrinkles when it is in repose, and thighs and breasts present an even sadder sight.

It is a pity that so few women realise in time that their bodies are more fragile than men's. This does not mean they cannot work hard or perform great feats of endurance, but where the actual flesh is concerned they are less durable. If every mother could teach her daughter this truth while she is still young there would be less miserable middle-aged women in the world.

Exercises are a great help in keeping slim and well, but exercise alone cannot work miracles if people persist in wrong diet and in eating to excess. Even yoga exercises, which are most effective of all due to their influence on the glands, will not really slim down a woman who regularly fills herself up with cakes, sweets and starches, nor save the health of one who destroys herself with excessive alcohol.

People often think that the practice of yoga means giving up all the food you like and becoming a freak eater, living on the most austere and miserable vegetarian diet. This is quite ridiculous, although as we have explained, a true yogi, or student seeking advanced spiritual development, must live on a restricted diet; but ordinary western householders, practising yoga for their health and well-being, are not obliged to make any drastic alteration in their eating habits, provided these are already sane and healthy.

Unfortunately, the diet of many people is not sane or healthy and in these cases yoga does suggest that changes should be made. So many ulcers, so much constipation, high blood-pressure, chronic indigestion, nervous tension and loss of looks and vitality are caused by wrong eating that there is obviously room for improvement.

What we eat and how we eat it can make or mar our lives, our health and our looks. Foolish eating affects everyone adversely, but especially women, who are so much more dependent than men on their appearance. As well as the loss of looks, the ruined figures and blotchy complexions caused by too much food and drink, there are usually bad psychological results, for these disfigurements are harder for a woman to carry off than they are for a man. Fat men are sometimes not unattractive in appearance, but most really fat women are aesthetically displeasing. They look years older than their age; they can never be chic or elegant, they must wear shapeless and depressing clothes and often these things affect their mental attitude. They develop an inferiority complex, a defensive attitude, hostility and jealousy towards more attractive women. They compensate for their unhappiness by overeating, which increases their troubles, and so a vicious circle is started.

Even in normal circumstances most people eat too much. As the body gets older it does not need so much food as when it is growing, or engaged in youthful activities . . . running, jumping, skipping, swimming and dancing . . . activities which quickly burn up the food consumed; yet it is common for people to eat more and more as they get older. Perhaps it is because with age their economic circumstances improve and they can afford to eat more richly and more lavishly;

perhaps it is because they have substituted food for other pleasures which they can no longer enjoy; whatever the reason, they eat twice as much as they did in youth, and since they take less than half the amount of exercise they soon become typical victims of prosperity . . . fat, bloated, red-faced, full of chronic ailments. It does not hurt the average healthy adult to cut down on food. This was plainly shown in England during the war when people lived for years on a greatly restricted diet under conditions of intense strain and anxiety, yet retained a reasonable standard of health.

So much is now being written in the popular Press about diet and nutrition that there is no longer any excuse for ignorance; but an unbalanced attitude is as bad as indifference and women who rush from one diet to another, always changing and experimenting, will not achieve much beyond indigestion. The only thing to do is to find a diet that suits you and stick to it if you want to stay healthy and slim.

A very common female practice is to indulge a weakness for sweets and cakes and then starve for several days in an effort to restore the balance. This is very foolish, for it upsets the stomach, gives a drawn expression to the face and results in bad temper, caused by an outraged and unsatisfied digestive system. It is very hard for some women to refrain from sweet things, especially housewives who are fond of cooking, and it is not made easier for them by the women's magazines which, publishing slimming diets on one page, devote sections of the paper to recipes and enticing colour-photographs of things guaranteed to destroy anyone's figure; but restraint is the only satisfactory way to reduce and stay slim.

You must cut out cakes and sweets, white bread and white sugar, which are bad for both figure and teeth; you must avoid fats and cream and chocolate, which are also bad for the liver; and you must try to give up having little snacks at all hours, eating three meals a day and nothing in between. This might sound rather forbidding and it may require some self-control, but many women have proved that it can be done, and the happiness that results, the satisfaction of having a slim figure, of being able to wear elegant clothes, is really worth the effort and will give far more lasting pleasure than the few coffee parties you have had to forgo.

Everyone needs sugar in some form, but if you can take honey, say at breakfast, you will find that your craving for cakes and sweets will diminish and even disappear, and if you eat fruit and dried fruit you will get all the sweetness your body needs without having to fill your teacup with white sugar.

Women who are not specially concerned with weight, but who wish to stay young, healthy and full of vitality as long as possible, should also work out a well-balanced diet to suit themselves and try to keep to it. It is not proposed to write a dissertation on nutrition here, for there is plenty of material available on this subject, but it is suggested that in the matter of eating the three main principles should be selectivity, moderation and mastication. Choose your food carefully and wisely; do not eat too much of it and always chew it properly, for the right food, improperly chewed, is just as indigestible as the wrong food.

If you have been eating meat in moderation all your life there is no need to suddenly become a rigid vegetarian unless for health reasons. Such a complete change may even upset the system if undertaken too abruptly; on the other hand, there is no doubt that a good vegetarian diet is often more beneficial than destructive, for many people eat too much meat, often—as in Australia—as much as three times a day, which in a warm climate is foolish and even dangerous. Replace some of your meat meals with fish, cheese and eggs. Cheese is best eaten uncooked, but there are endless ways of cooking fish and eggs so that no one need complain of monotony.

If you are not worried about your weight, and if you can drink milk, which is a food as well as a drink; and if you do not like milk, or if it makes you too fat, take yoghurt or buttermilk. Both are excellent foods, and even if you begin by disliking them the taste can be cultivated, up to the point of enjoyment. Try to learn to eat yoghurt without sugar, taking it alone or on vegetables as a sauce.

Eat as much fresh fruit as you can afford, where possible unpeeled, after careful washing. If your system is inclined to be acid be moderate with such acid fruits as lemons, oranges and pineapples.

Eat also plenty of green vegetables and where vegetables in general are concerned take them raw whenever feasible. Do not peel or cut them and leave them for hours in water, as some women do, changing the water before cooking and thus throwing away their most valuable properties. From the health point of view steaming is the best way to cook vegetables but some people complain this is dull and monotonous. Whatever method you choose, they must not be overcooked and in boiling them use a minimum of water, not throwing it away afterwards but keeping it for stock or gravy.[1]

You should try to eat some kind of salad every day, either a simple green salad of lettuce, with or without French dressing, or a mixture of fruit and vegetables. In certain circles a salad consists of a damp exhausted lettuce leaf, a slice of beetroot, a slice of tomato and a slice of cucumber, perhaps embellished with some cold tinned peas and potato mayonnaise, even a pile of finely grated carrot, like wet sawdust, or a piece of tinned pineapple. This sort of thing is unlikely to attract anyone who enjoys good eating, and it is extremely monotonous even to those who are used to it; yet salads offer great possibilities for the exercise of imagination and require very little apparatus to produce. Raw vegetables need not be limited to lettuce, cucumber and tomato; carrots, cabbage, celery, onions and green vegetables can be

1. In this we can learn from the Chinese, who barely half-cook their vegetables.

grated up and used. A coarse shredder is far better for vegetables than a fine one, for it leaves them sufficiently intact to retain some kind of texture, and by experimenting with combinations you will not only produce good salads from the point of nutrition but dishes that are appetising and visually attractive.

We have given the recipe at the end of this chapter for a salad we evolved ourselves: a combination of raw fruit, vegetables and nuts which has been eaten with enjoyment by vegetarians, meat eaters and *bon viveurs*, and which is not hard or expensive to make.

To be a vegetarian does not mean that food must be tasteless and depressing. It is not the absence of meat that makes some vegetarian diets so unpalatable but the absence of imagination in the cook, for a poor cook can spoil any kind of food, vegetarian or otherwise. If you can learn to treat vegetables as the French treat them, as items worthy of individual attention and not just a tasteless background for meat, your attitude to vegetarian food might change.

Women who are troubled with indigestion should give up fried foods, heated-up foods, pastries and meat cooked to the consistency of leather. They must avoid bolting their food and should try to find time, especially at breakfast, to sit down and eat properly. Breakfast need only be a light meal (fruit, cereal, yoghurt, honey—whatever you wish), but it should be eaten in peace, not taken standing up at the dressing-table or gulped down as you run for the bus. This is the surest way to ruin your digestion and spoil your whole day. Try also to eat your evening meal in peace in a pleasant atmosphere. A large hot dinner late at night, when nerves and stomach are tired from the day's work, is quite bad enough, but if it is eaten in a noisy or discordant atmosphere, if it is accompanied by family bickering or depressing conversation, it will result in indigestion, nervous tension and insomnia.

The preparation and presentation of all food is important (and especially so in vegetarian cooking). Colour, texture, serving-dishes, the table setting, all influence the appetite and digestion. It is not a question of elaborate or expensive appointments but rather of understanding how to make things look attractive and palatable. Very simple food, garnished with parsley, mint or lettuce, served in a pleasant setting, with fresh flowers on the table, is far more enjoyable and beneficial to the digestion than a pretentious affair badly presented; while those damp and dreary concoctions we have mentioned, served up as salads, those sloppy boiled vegetables which have lain for hours in cooking water that has absorbed away their life-blood, are not only tasteless and aesthetically repulsive but almost useless as nourishment.

Constipation

You cannot expect to be well if you are constipated, yet many women who spend much time and money on their faces will go on from week to week with a system that is clogged up and poisoned. As the body gets older its natural powers of evacuation become weaker unless they are developed by proper exercise, until the system finally reaches a state where it is chronically contaminated. There may be a bowel movement every day but the victim is still constipated because she has incomplete elimination and as a result she feels tired, depressed, liverish with headaches and backaches and other vague feelings of malaise.

Helping the eliminative system does not mean stirring it up with purgatives or chemical laxatives but rather by such natural means as proper diet and the re-education of abdominal muscles. The stomach contractions described on pages 147–50 (*Uddiyana* and *Nauli*), practised every morning while the stomach is empty, will help to cure constipation, and if a glass of warm slightly salted water is taken beforehand the effect will be laxative. Relaxation, exercise, a diet in which fruit and vegetables replace heavy starches will also help, and the following *asanas* will speed up results:

Asanas: Uddiyana (page 149); *Nauli* (page 150); Fish (page 143); Cobra (page 142); Locust (page 143); Headstand (page 135); Shoulderstand (page 131); Half-shoulderstand (page 133); Archer (page 140); Spinal Twist (page 141); *Yoga-mudra* (page 154); Supine Pelvic (page 145); Head-to-knee (page 139).

Fasting

Fasting is not starving, as many people seem to think, and if it is done in the proper way it can be beneficial to a system full of impurities. We have mentioned the foolishness of skipping meals to compensate for over-indulgence, but a day of fasting is quite a different matter. It helps the body to throw off poisons in nature's own way, and if you can arrange to do it on a day when you do not have to work or go out or exert yourself physically it will do you no harm. Yoga students sometimes go on longer fasts, for three or four days, even for a week or more, but for the average busy woman with a job or household to look after a one-day fast is more practical and convenient.

During the fast take only water, and rest as much as you can. Go to bed early and if you can, arrange to be alone and keep silent all day, not answering the telephone or making any calls. Conserve all your vital energy, even your voice, and next morning you will feel remarkably refreshed.

Fasting for purification is usually accompanied by an enema at the end of the day, to help the body get rid of its impurities.

The water-fast could be replaced by a fruit-juice fast, in which fruit and vegetable juices are taken; or if you can afford to lose weight you could limit yourself to a one-fruit diet for several days. On these days eat only the same kind of fruit . . . all apples or all oranges or whatever suits you best. If you want to lose weight do not imitate the pupil who chose bananas as her fruit. She was disappointed to find that at the end of the third day she had lost no weight at all but gained acute indigestion; nor should you emulate another woman who took her fruit-juice fast on the day she was playing competition tennis, and who, after an all-day tournament played in intense heat, wondered why she felt giddy and exhausted. Use common sense and discretion and you will find a short fast entirely beneficial, unless you are already underweight, in which case fasting should not be practised.

Liquids

If you can afford it, buy a fruit-juice extractor, and if you cannot afford it try to give up something else so you can still buy it. It is one of the most important items in the kitchen of a woman who wants to keep her health, figure and complexion, and the money you spend on it will be saved from cosmetic bills. One of its greatest advantages is that it enables you to drink combinations of fruit or vegetables which would otherwise be difficult to make. Such combinations as apple and orange, tomato and celery, tomato and parsley, tomato and capsicum, strawberry and lemon, carrot and lemon, carrot and apple, apple and blackberry, are all worth trying, and many other combinations of two or more fruit and/or vegetables could be worked out.

Milk, as we have already said, is an excellent drink, if you can take it, being also a food in itself. For this reason it must be 'chewed' before being swallowed, and if it is gulped down it will become very indigestible. Buttermilk is also a remarkable drink, satisfying, digestible and nourishing, and harmless where weight is concerned.

A very pleasant drink for hot weather, which is also satisfying and sustaining, is the Turkish drink called *ayran*. It is made with half yoghurt, half water, with a little salt, shaken up together, and is best drunk cold.

At one time there was a belief that water was fattening, but most people now realise this is a fallacy. Water, in itself, contains no calories; it can be fattening only when it is drunk in excess with meals, when it has the same effects as any other fluid taken in the same way. In itself it is the best and healthiest of all drinks, and the remedy for many ailments. It flushes the kidneys, washes out poisons, clears the complexion and purifies the blood. It is cheap and available to most people in the west.

Alcohol and tobacco

Yoga has no moralistic attitude towards alcohol. A true yogi does not drink it because he knows that it is a form of poison and when taken to excess will impair his health and prevent his spiritual advancement. The word 'intoxication' is self-explanatory, coming from the word toxin or poison.

For the average householder there is only one safe rule to follow. Yoga teaches that if you are master of yourself and your habits nothing can harm you; but unfortunately few of us are complete masters of ourselves and where there is a danger of being overcome it is wisest to try to avoid the evil. However, since this is not always practical in modern western life, where sometimes social obligations make it difficult to completely abstain, the only thing is to try to cultivate self-control, to practise moderation in drinking as well as in eating.

The same may be said about smoking. It is a form of poison that can only cause harm if indulged to excess, and no one expecting full benefits from breathing exercises would inhale tobacco. A real yogi would not smoke; but as with alcohol, the choice is with yourself. If you are one of the few who can take an occasional drink or cigarette and leave it at that, then there is no reason why you should not do so if you wish.

To sum up: it is possible to keep your health and vitality without increasing weight if a sensible diet is followed. This diet should include meat, if desired, in moderation; fish; eggs; cheese; milk or milk products such as yoghurt or buttermilk; plenty of fruit, vegetables—raw whenever possible—wholemeal bread, fruit juices and water.

Women worried about their weight must cut out little snacks, coffee parties with the girls, female lunches and teas where everyone eats too much. If you are fond of cooking, or are obliged for some reason to cook rich and fattening meals, try to stop yourself from tasting as you work; try also to break yourself of a habit common to many young mothers . . . of finishing up the children's puddings and sweet cakes; try to give up sugar in tea and if you cannot take it unsweetened take honey. Try to substitute honey for sugar wherever you can.

If you have reduced and want to keep your weight in check get a calorie chart and study the calorie content of different foods, adjusting your meals accordingly. If you are very much overweight ask your doctor for a reducing diet, and do not experiment with slimming drugs or freak diets that promise to reduce you overnight. They are not worth the risk to health and looks; and it is possible to reduce quite safely if you make up your mind.

Fruit and vegetable salad

Using a coarse grater—a French *mandolin* if you can get one—grate up the following:

One carrot; one apple; one or two sticks of celery; several radishes; a small quantity of red cabbage. Mix them together and add a handful of fresh chopped parsley, some dried fruit . . . sultanas, raisins, candied peel, etc. . . . some unblanched almonds (or other nuts) previously roasted in the oven. Mix a French dressing of oil, lemon-juice, a pinch of salt and brown sugar or honey to taste, and pour over the salad. If you like sprinkle some chopped nuts or grape-nut cereal over the top.

The appeal of this salad is its mixture of flavours, sweet and sharp, and its crisp and nutty texture. You can vary the ingredients as you choose, so long as you keep the crisp character, which will be spoilt if you add wet things like tomatoes, pineapples and oranges. If you are making the salad in quantity, for keeping in the refrigerator, as some women do, do not include the almonds or dressing, which should both be added just before eating. The almonds will become soft if kept with the vegetables, and the whole salad lose its special texture if soaked too long in dressing.

6

Physical and mental hygiene

Body hygiene

A daily bath or shower should be taken by everyone who has access to facilities and whose health does not forbid the practice. Climatic conditions should make no difference to personal cleanliness, though women living in cold countries often think it is not necessary to bath each day. The skin of people in the tropics is constantly exposed to the air, and in most cases is frequently washed, for comfort if not for health, but in cold countries the body is wrapped up in heavy clothes which, absorbing stale emanations given off by the skin itself, unventilated, the pores clogged with discharged impurities, becomes sickly and unhealthy. This condition is bad in anyone but especially so in women, whose bodies should be kept always fresh and fragrant.

In some western countries, and particularly in the cities, conditions do not encourage the taking of daily baths, and those who do take them often do so at night. This is better than taking no bath at all, but unfortunately they are usually taken too hot and too prolonged, with enervating and damaging results. Other people wash their bodies with cologne instead of water, and though this is, of course, a method of cleaning, it cannot give the feeling of freshness and stimulation of a bath or shower, and in time the cologne has a very drying effect on the skin.

Even better than a morning bath is a warm shower, followed by a cold one if you can stand it; but it is not suggested that you should suddenly start taking cold showers in winter if you are not used to them. Apart from causing chronic cold feet and chilblains in people with bad circulations they can be a shock to the heart, though for normal healthy people they are a refreshing and stimulating practice.

Whether it is a bath or shower, the water should not be too hot. It is not only exhausting and enervating but is very bad for the skin, drying up the natural oils and often causing unsightly blemishes. Women with sensitive skins can develop ugly broken capillaries on the legs or on the body through constantly soaking in very hot water. A favourite habit with some women is to read in the bath for long periods, replenishing the hot water as it cools off, and though there may be truth in their claim that this is the only time they can get peace and quiet to read, the fact is the blood, drawn suddenly to the surface of the skin and kept there by the heat of the water, can cause these disfigurements that are either permanent or extremely expensive to remove. Anyone who goes to the beach in summer knows how unsightly this sort of thing can be.

This can also happen to the skin of the face, and people who recommend plunging it into hot then into icy cold water are responsible for a great deal of damage to delicate complexions, for only a few skins can stand such treatment. The same may be said for those who advocate scrubbing the face hard with a brush. It is, of course, essential to keep the face clean but not to destroy it in the process, and women with dry or fragile skins cannot afford to treat them so roughly.

Soap. Many soaps have a very drying effect on the skin and it is always advisable to use an oily type unless your skin is abnormally oily. Cheap soap full of strong soda will eventually spoil the average complexion.

Colognes and talc powder. Good colognes and body essences are very pleasant and refreshing after a bath, but they have a definite drying effect on the skin and should not be used too lavishly or too frequently. Spray your skin perfume inside elbows and wrists, not drenching yourself all over as many women do. Talcum powder is perhaps better, but it too has a drying effect and also clogs the pores.

Oil baths. From time to time it is a good idea to take an oil bath, especially at the change of the seasons when the skin has become dried or cracked by winter winds or hot summer sun. After a warm bath or shower, while the pores of the skin are still open, rub yourself all over with slightly warmed oil . . . olive oil if possible, or any other you prefer; then if you can spare the time wrap yourself in towels, lie down and relax for a while.

Sun-baths and air-baths. A healthy sun-tan can be very attractive, but a skin that has been burnt raw is quite hideous. Though aware of this, many women seem unable to relate it to themselves, refusing to accept the fact that only certain types of skin will tan safely and evenly, and that, for the rest, no amount of sunbathing will ever result in anything but red and peeling noses or scarlet arms and legs.

Even those who tan easily should use discretion, for sunbaking for long periods in the hottest part of the day is not only harmful to the health but can destroy the skin itself. A dried and wrinkled face, a red and leathery neck do not improve any woman's appearance, yet girls continue to invite these things by over-exposure to a hot sun, as they do in Australia, where sunbathing starts in childhood and where women age early.

Sunbathing in moderation is excellent, even necessary, being beneficial to the general health and appearance, soothing the nerves and replenishing vital energy; but when done to excess it saps the vitality, drugs the brain, ages the skin and often causes skin cancer.

Take your sun-baths gradually, and at the beginning of summer do not try to tan yourself too quickly. Like hot baths, a sudden violent dose of sun can cause unsightly blemishes on the legs.

Air-baths, which are taken lying in the shade or under trees, are also a pleasant and beneficial practice. If you have the necessary privacy take your air-bath without any clothes, otherwise do it in a swimming costume. Completely relax while letting the air refresh your skin, so often covered up and shut off from the life-giving properties in the atmosphere around us.

Teeth

Despite all the modern publicity given to dental care there are still many people who do not clean their teeth enough, or, if they do, clean them the wrong way. You should always clean your teeth before going to bed, to remove any scraps of food caught between them, and during the day, if possible after each meal. This is not such a nuisance as it sounds and can soon become a regular habit which not only keeps the teeth clean but helps to freshen the mouth and breath.

When cleaning the teeth do not brush from side to side, for this will not remove the food particles caught between the teeth but it will encourage the gums to recede. Teeth in the top jaw should be brushed downwards and the lower ones with an upward stroke. The same action should be used in massaging the gums with the finger, to prevent recession.

If you cannot clean your teeth at any time at least rinse out your mouth with salt water, swilling vigorously round the teeth and gums. Salt and water can also be used if you have no toothpaste, for though this gives a pleasant taste in the mouth, in itself it is not essential for cleaning the teeth. It is the action of the brush that is important.

Cleaning the tongue

An excellent custom not often practised in the west is cleaning the tongue. Once you have done it a couple of times you will wonder how you ever managed without it. In the east there are special attachments on toothbrushes to be used for this purpose but the same results can be achieved with a spoon.

Stand before a mirror and put out your tongue; then scrape it carefully with an inverted spoon, washing away the deposits as they are collected. This must be done in the morning before eating or drinking anything at all, otherwise all the impurities collected on the tongue during the night will be washed back into the system.

Gargling will also help to keep the mouth fresh and clean, but be sure not to use strong solutions or mouthwashes that can burn delicate membranes. Use a mild well-diluted antiseptic, or salt and warm water.

Inner cleanliness (see also page 81—constipation).
You must be clean inside as well as outside. Try to overcome any tendency to constipation by wise diet, exercise and the practice of stomach contractions, *Uddiyana* and *Nauli* (pages 149–50). These should be done every morning as soon as you get up, while the stomach is empty, and should become an indispensable part of your morning toilet. If you are pressed for time in the morning they can be done while you are under the shower or making-up your face.

If constipation persists, or if the bloodstream is contaminated by wrong diet, smoking or drinking, a day of fasting (see Chapter 5), followed by an enema, will help rid the system of impurities.

For complete cleanliness, according to yoga teaching, the rectum should be washed after a bowel movement. This custom, which is more common in the east than the west, should be included in the normal daily routine.

A vaginal douche of warm salty water is another necessary part of hygiene in women (see Chapter 4).

Dress
Modern dress is so sane and healthy that the old warnings about tight corsets and garters no longer have much meaning. However, high-heeled shoes continue to bring abuse from health authorities, and women who have been wearing shoes with pointed toes in recent years are now complaining that their feet are becoming deformed.

To most women high heels are more than an article of dress; they are an important aid to self-confidence, therefore few will give them up, despite warnings that they harm the health, ruin the carriage, deform the feet, cause bunions, corns and prolapses. The only thing we can suggest is to go without shoes as much as possible, wherever you can . . . at the beach, at home, in the country.

Varicose veins are encouraged by tight or high-heeled shoes, particularly in hot weather. This condition can be improved, even cured, by regular practice of the inverted poses (pages 131–7).

Mental hygiene

No matter what efforts a woman makes with her physical appearance they will be wasted if her mental attitude is not right. Beauty of figure, complexion and dress all lose their appeal if a woman is bored, tense or disagreeable; while plain and dowdy women often hold attention and admiration through magnetism, vitality or sweetness of expression.

This is not an empty statement but a sober fact, obvious to anyone familiar with aimless society women who live only for themselves. There is nothing so depressing and unattractive as a gathering of physically beautiful, well-dressed women whose faces and conversations express only greed, spite, discontent of the ruthless drive of competition.

Some women are born philosophical but others have to strive to achieve this state, to overcome such

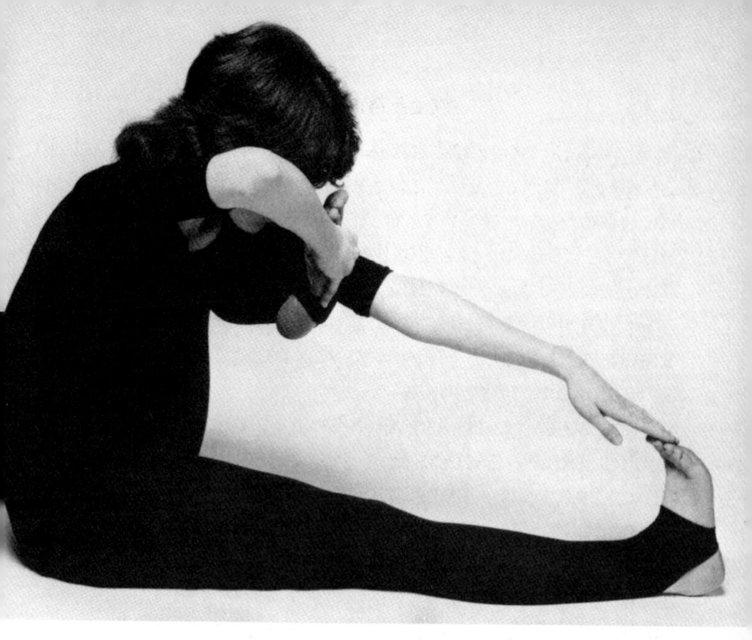

Plate 1 Archer

Plate 2 *Savasana,* Pose of Complete Rest

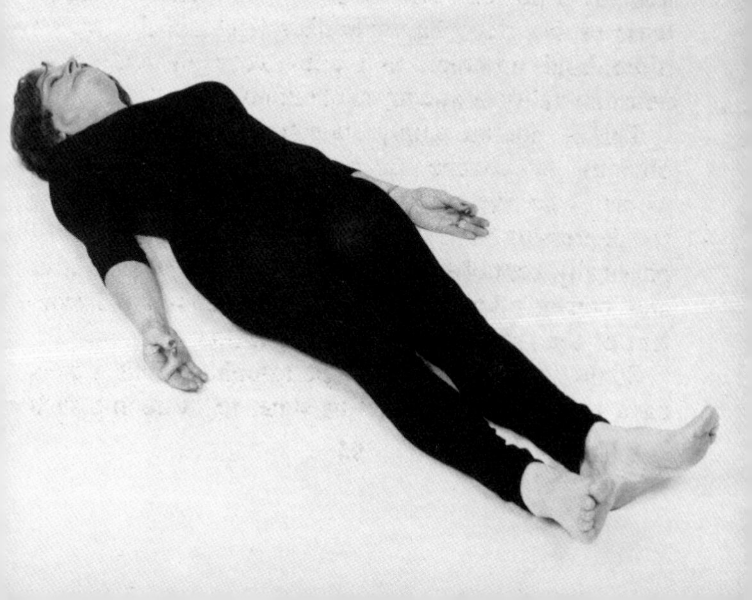

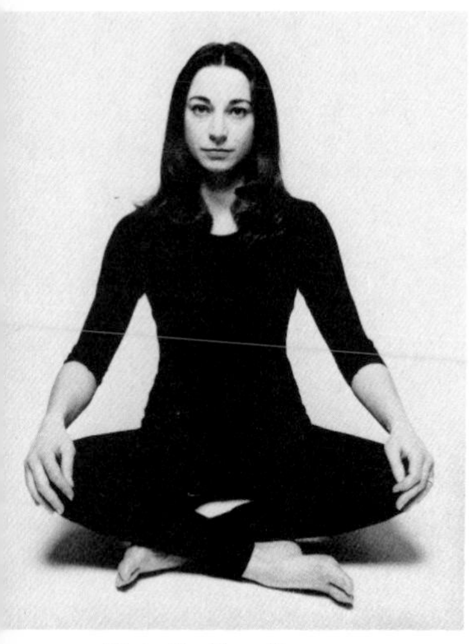

Plate 3 Easy Pose (simple cross-legged).

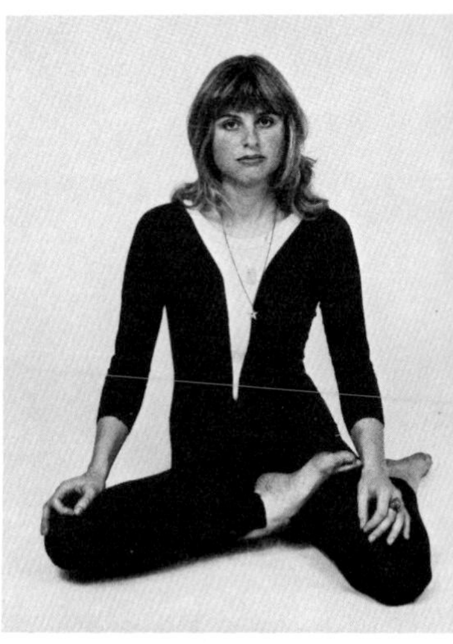

Plate 4 Pose of a Hero

Plate 5 Pose of an Adept

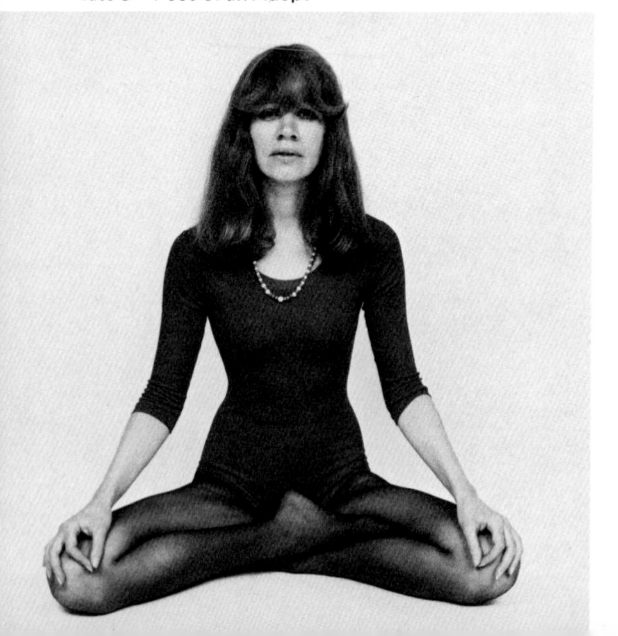

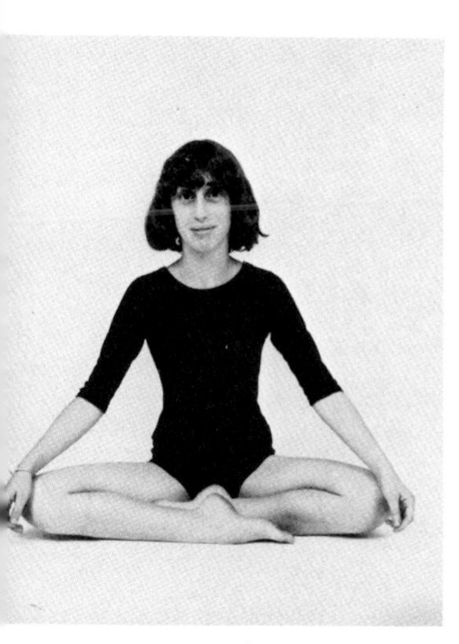

Plate 6 Free Pose

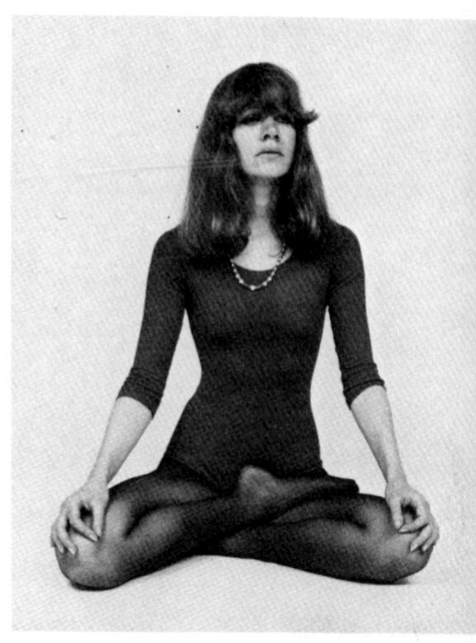

Plate 7 Half-Lotus

Plate 8 Lotus Position

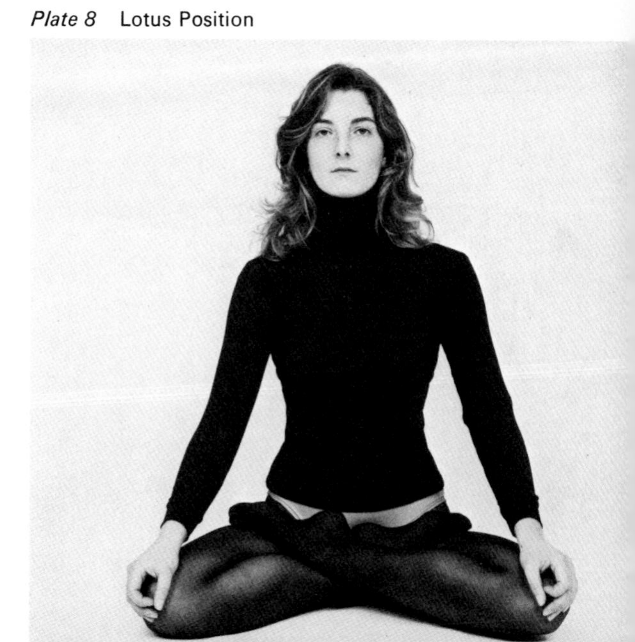

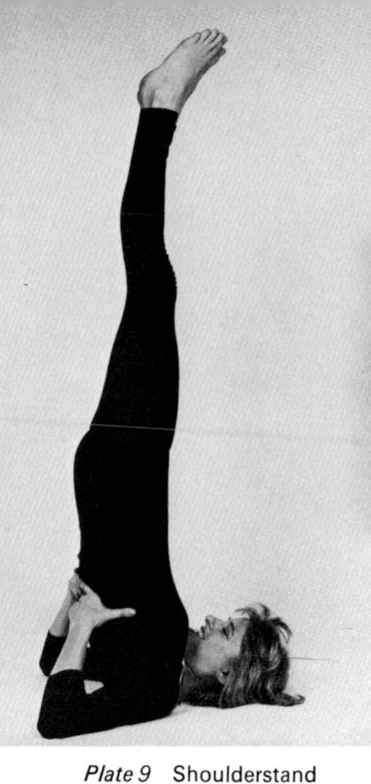

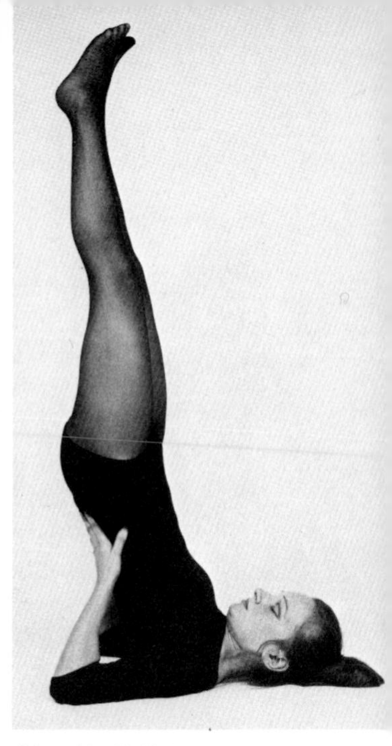

Plate 9 Shoulderstand

Plate 10 Half-shoulderstand

Plate 11 Triangular Pose

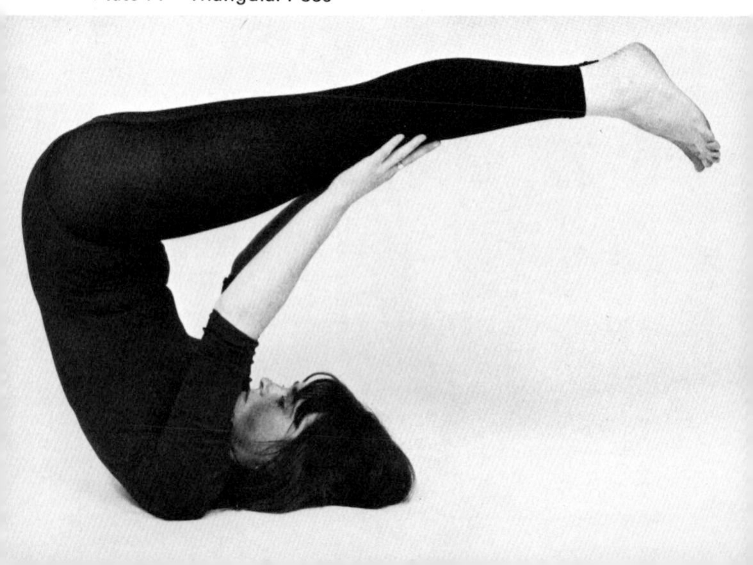

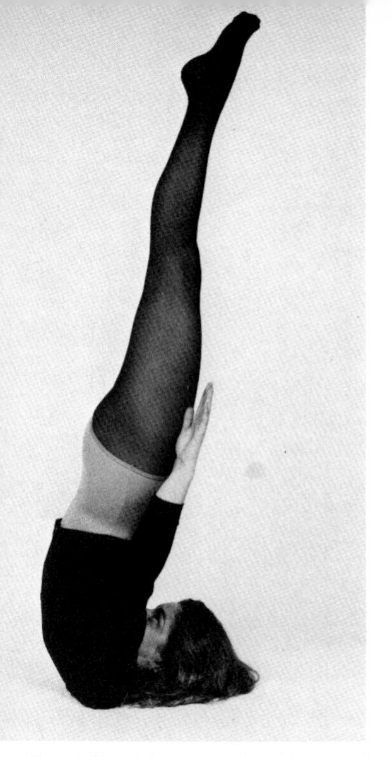

Plate 12 Balancing Shoulderstand

Plate 13 Choking Pose

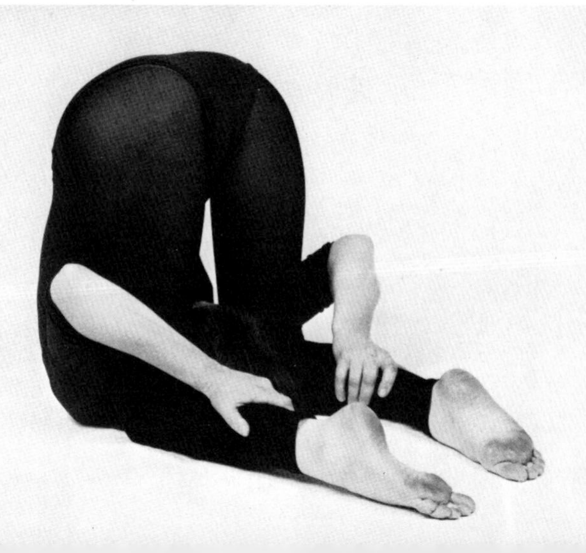

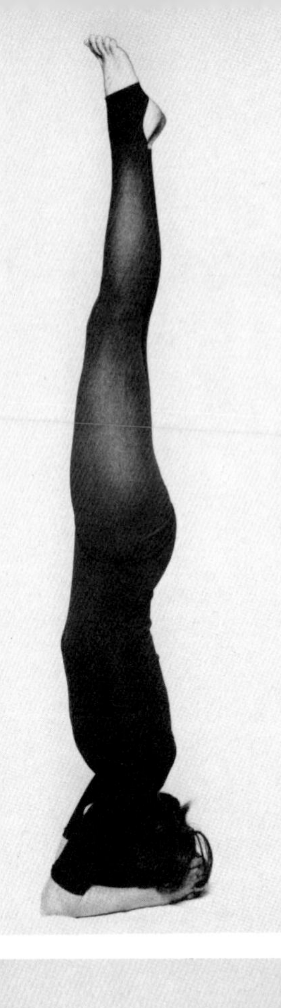

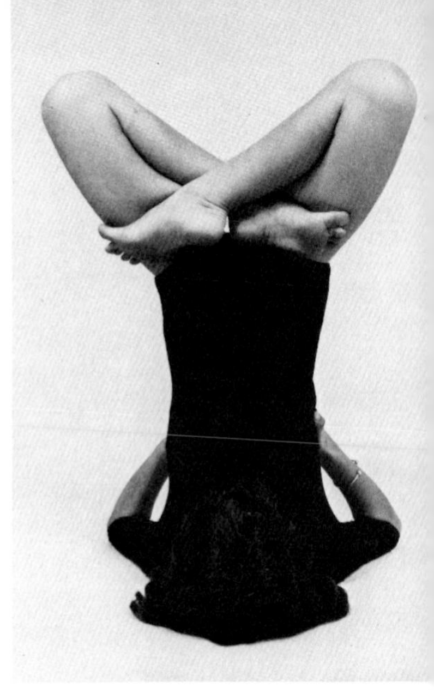

Plate 15 **Bound shoulderstand**

Plate 14 Headstand

Plate 16 Plough

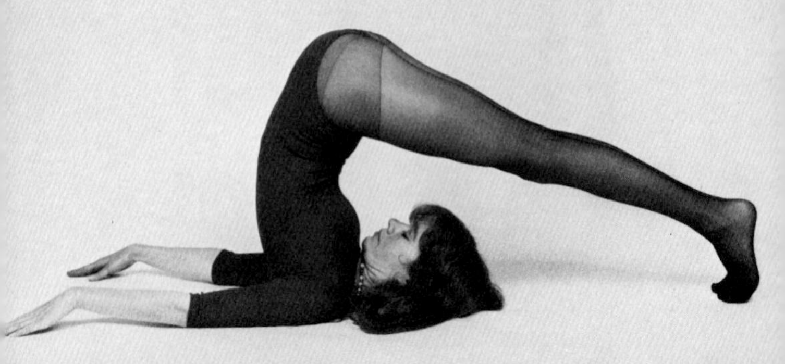

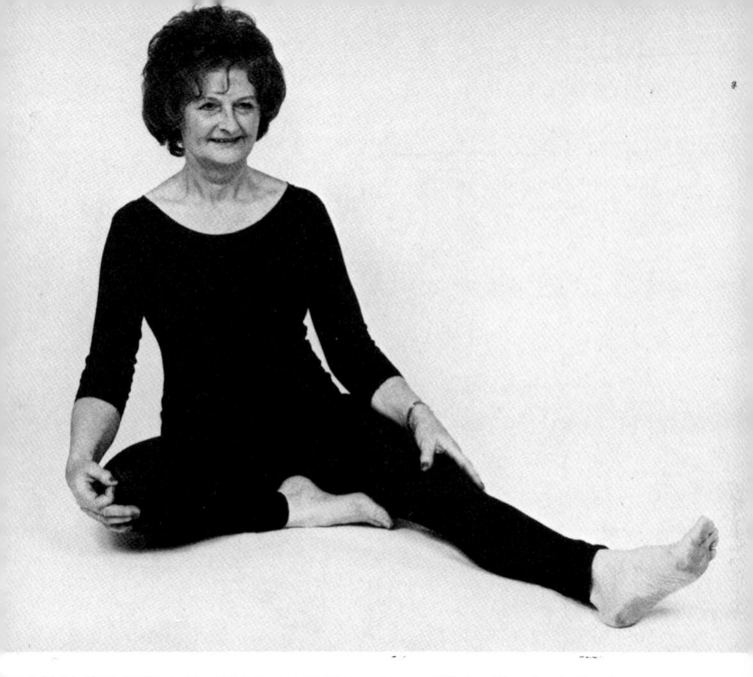

Plate 17 Arch Gesture

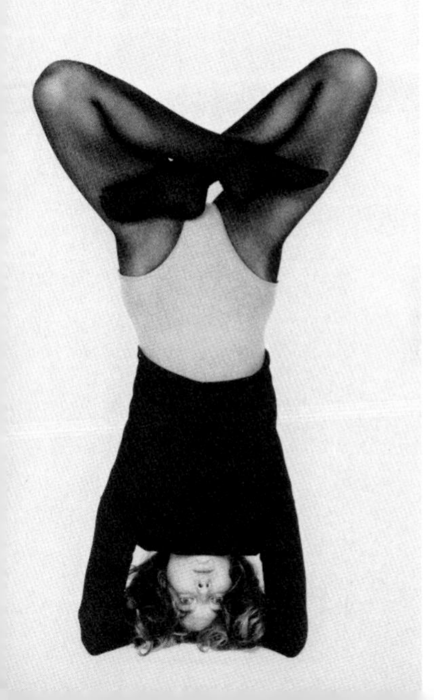

Plate 18
Bound Headstand

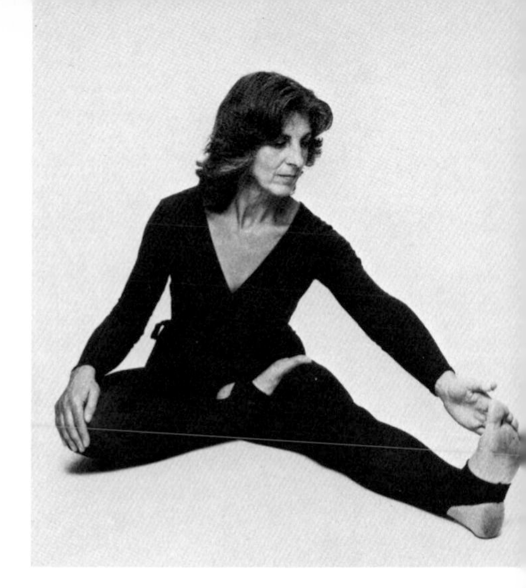

Plate 19
Variation of
Arch Gesture

Plate 20
Yoga Spinal Twist

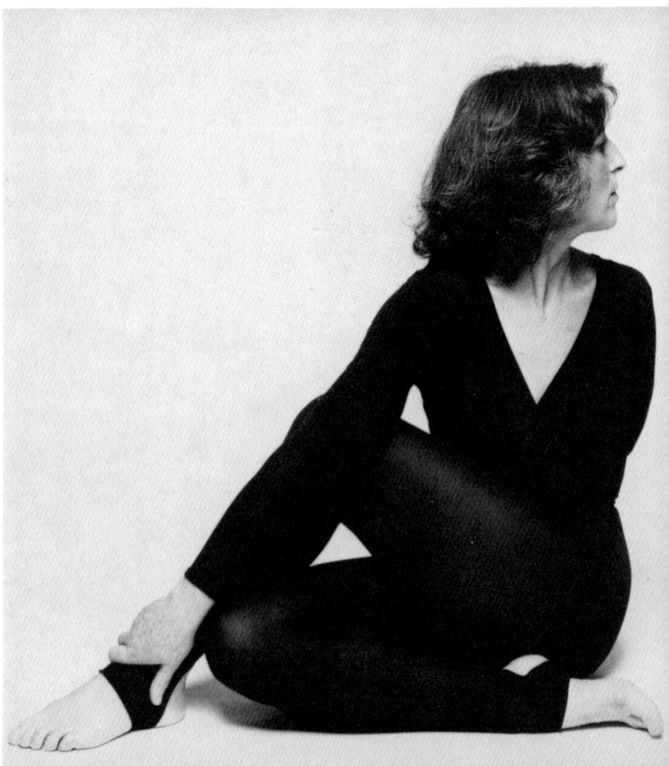

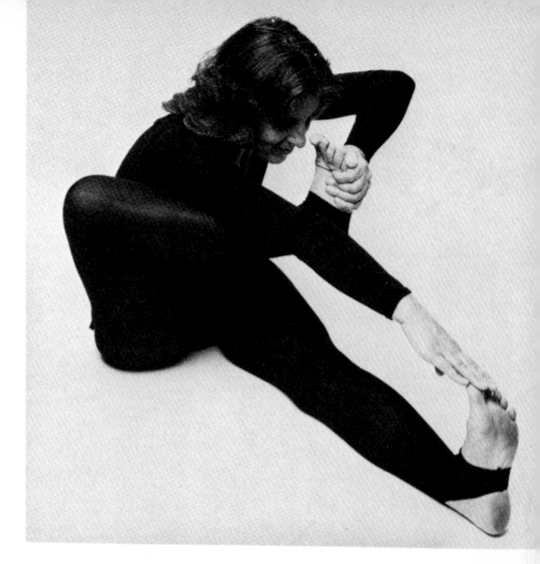

Plate 21 Archer

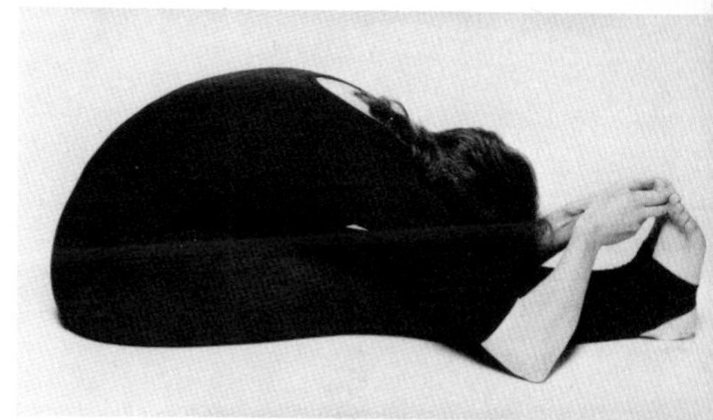

Plate 22
Head-to-knee
Pose

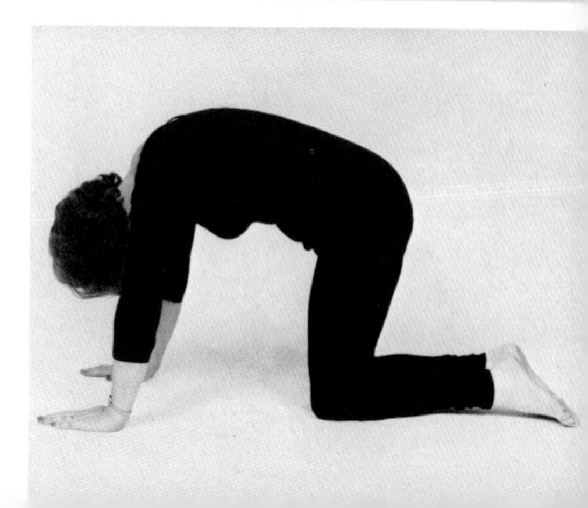

Plate 23
Pose of a Cat

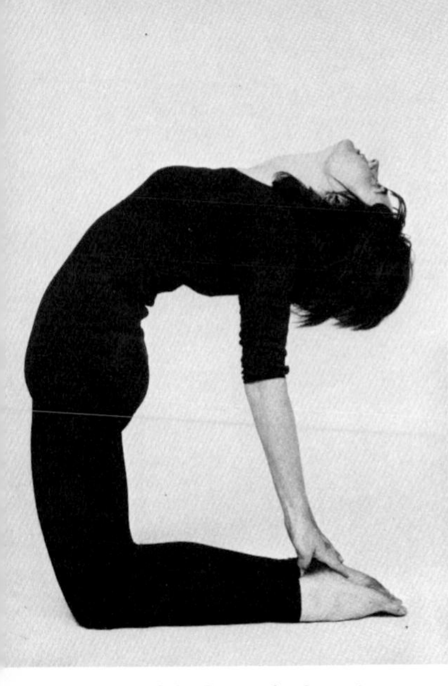

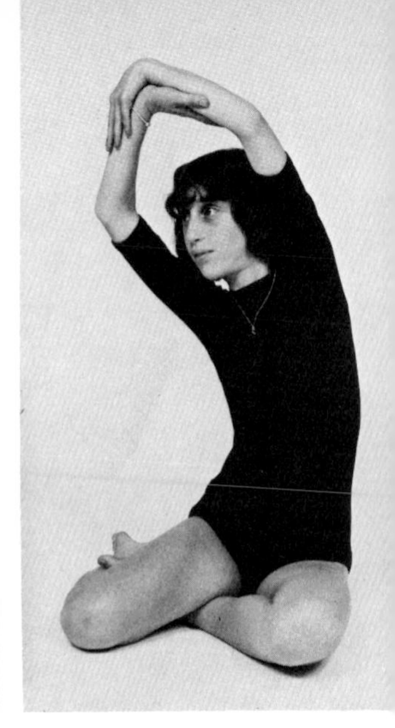

Plate 24 Pose of a Camel

Plate 25 Sideways Swing

Plate 26 Cobra

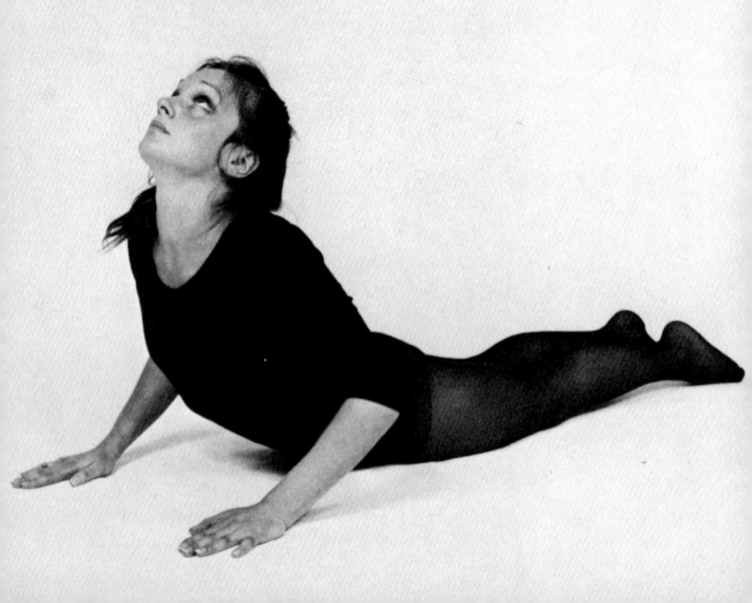

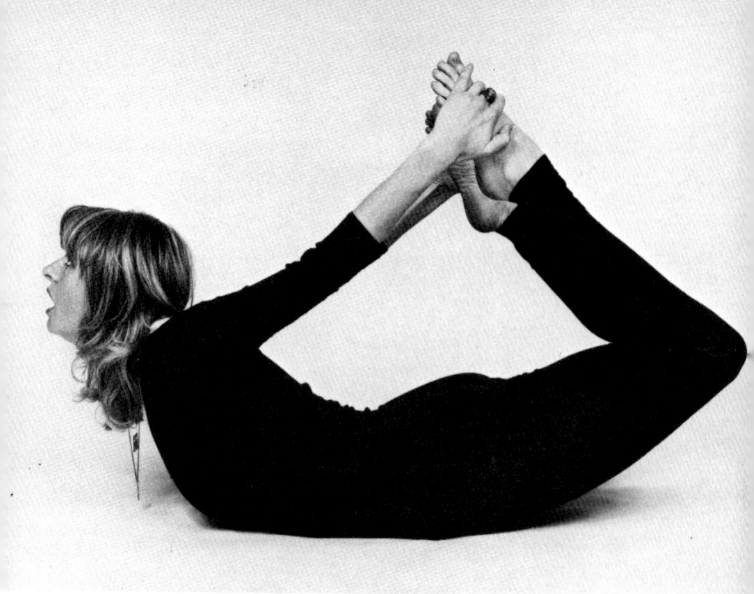

Plate 27 Bow

Plate 28 Wheel

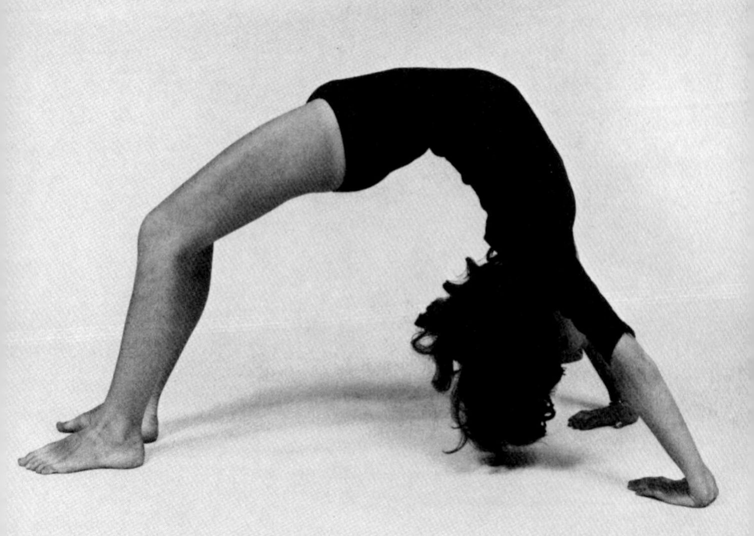

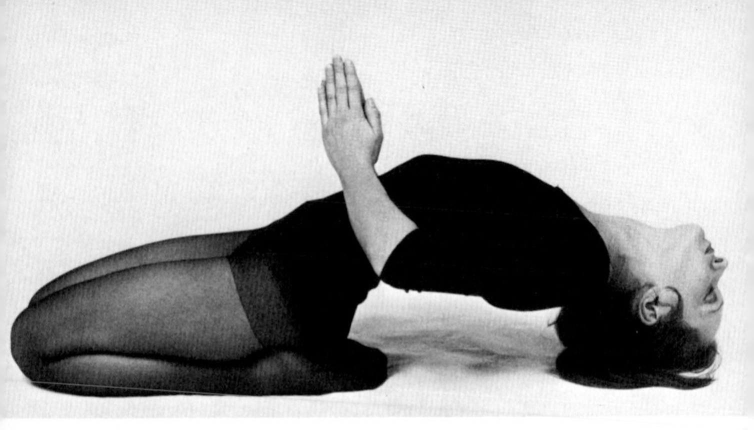

Plate 29 Supine Pelvic

Plate 30 Locust

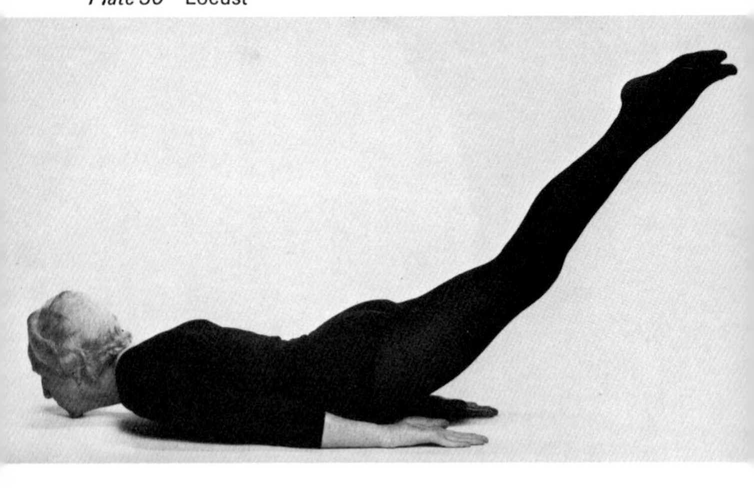

Plate 31 Fish

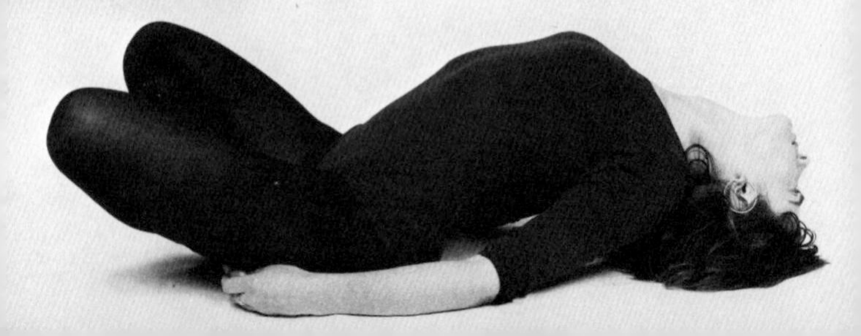

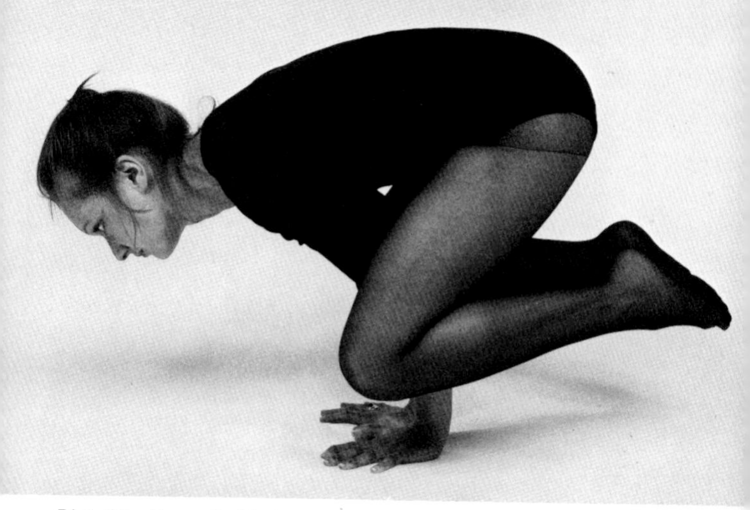

Plate 32 Pose of a Bird

Plate 33 Pose of a Raven

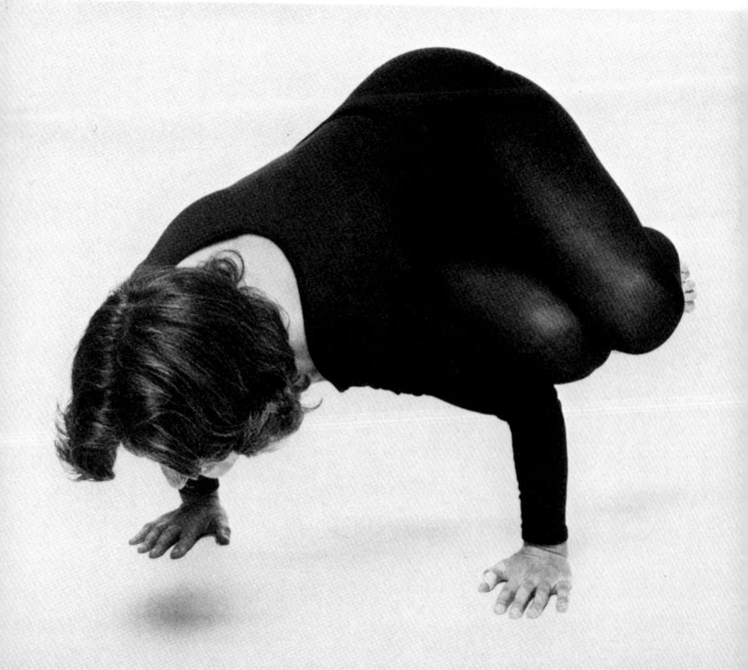

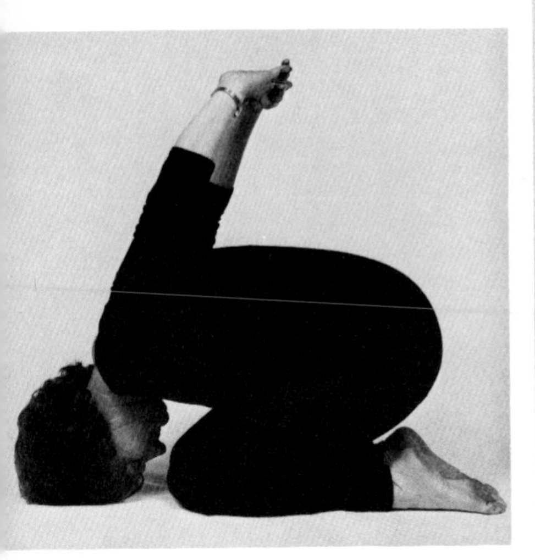

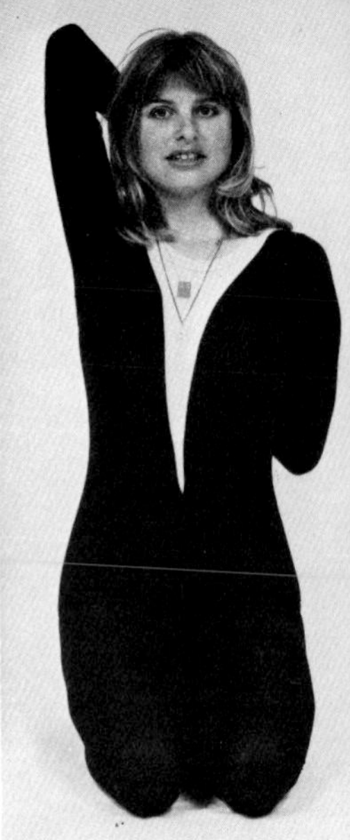

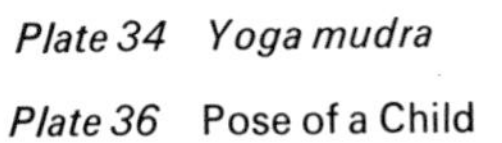

Plate 34 *Yoga mudra*

Plate 35 Head of a Cow

Plate 36 Pose of a Child

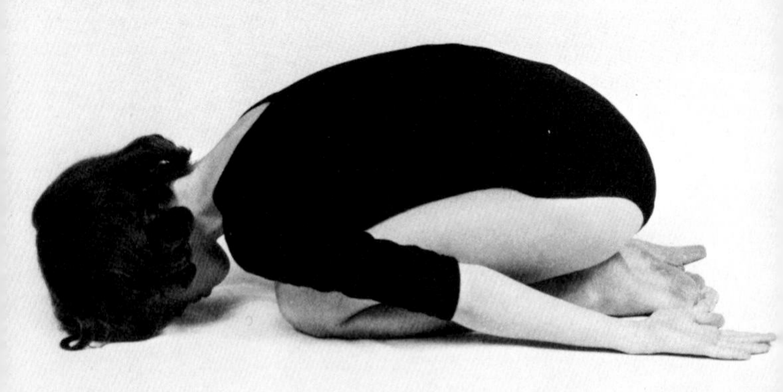

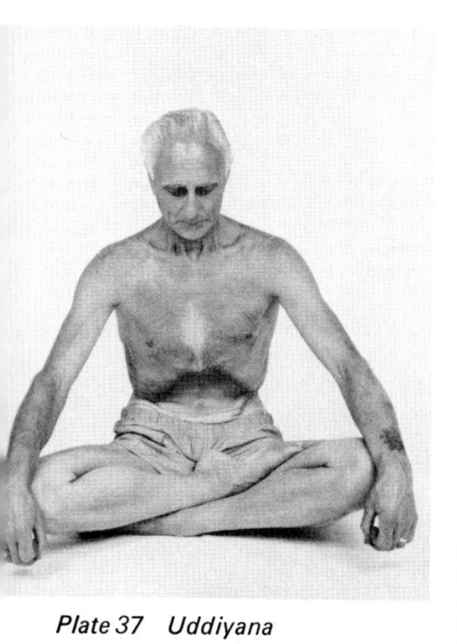

Plate 37 Uddiyana

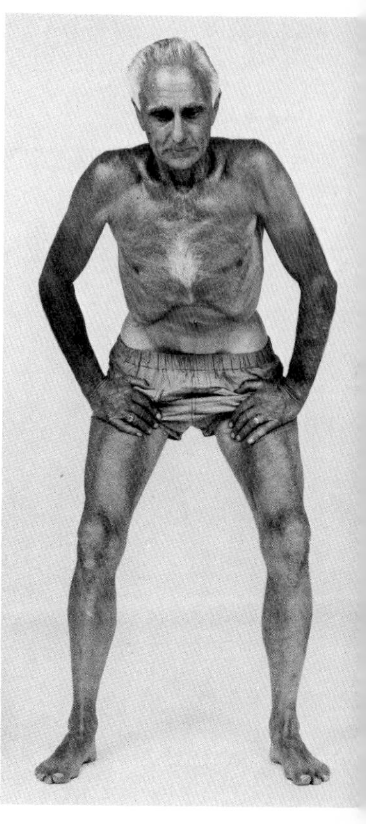

Plate 38 Nauli

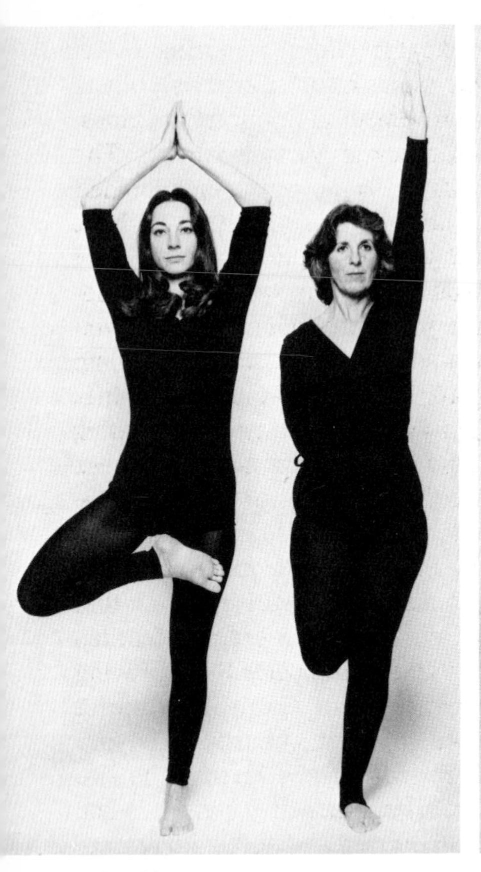

Plate 39
Tree and variation of Tree

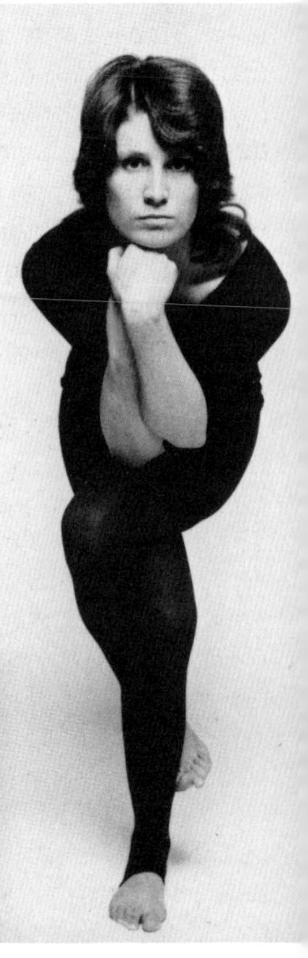

Plate 40
Eagle Pose

destructive emotions as envy, acquisitiveness, bitterness. Many never make the effort, preferring to remain miserable rather than help themselves; others regard talk of self-improvement as insincere or pious, tinged with the complacency of Victorian tracts. The truth, however, is that it is not just high-minded nonsense but plain common sense on the earthiest level. If, for example, you are eaten up by jealousy you are miserable; you become possessive, demanding, angry, suspicious; you want to hurt people, you never feel secure. You lie awake at night worrying; you nag and complain; you picture absurd things that may never happen and you end up by alienating everyone, not only those you hate but those you love. These emotions not only destroy your rest and age your face but also carve upon it an unmistakable expression that repels people even before you speak.

How do you overcome these negative things that spoil your life? How can you stop worrying, fearing, suspecting and hating? In the first place by improving your physical condition, and particularly the state of the glands which have so much influence on your outlook (see Chapter 2); secondly, by learning how to relax; and finally by persistent mental exercises. When the glands are working properly and the nerves are relaxed you will automatically become more optimistic and philosophical. You give up worrying and take life as it comes. But these benefits, excellent though they are, are only half the solution. To really triumph over yourself you must turn them into positive assets through the development of the mind.

Mental exercises are not easy and there is no point in pretending they are. There may be a long and discouraging struggle before any kind of results are achieved and it is easy to slip back and give up halfway. To the women who dismiss these exercises as useless or ridiculous, to those materialists who can believe in nothing that cannot be touched or seen with the physical eye, the only reply is 'Why not try and see what happens?' There is nothing to lose, and everything to gain.

The first thing to do is to get command of your mind, to discipline it to complete obedience. Many people never really have control of their mind at all; it flits about from one thing to another like a butterfly, and when they try to concentrate they find thoughts rushing through it like trains through a railway station; but if you are prepared to work at it you can control both mind and thoughts, for mental powers, like the muscles of the body, can be developed and strengthened by exercise. If will-power is never used it atrophies; if courage—moral or physical—is never exercised it fades away; and so with the powers of imagination and concentration.

Start your exercises in a simple way. Find a quiet place where you will not be disturbed and sit down in any comfortable cross-legged position. Sitting with back and neck in one straight line, close your eyes, rest the hands on the knees, or loosely clasped on your crossed legs, and commence your deep, slow breathing. Let the first exercise be a complete concentration on the process of breathing, to such an extent that you are almost unconscious of your physical body. This will help to calm your mind and every nervous centre. (Yoga teaches that by mastering this exercise you could deal with such minor maladies as headache, toothache, backache, etc., much more successfully than by taking powders or sedatives.)

See how you progress with this breathing and when you are satisfied try to attain complete stillness of mind. Remember that when the mind is completely stilled it is at its most receptive. This breathing exercise is the traditional beginning of meditation, whether directed towards self-realisation or used for some other purpose. (Meditation is not exclusively used for self-realisation but is also a method of contemplating any philosophical idea or even one's own personal problems.)

Usually, at first, the whole thing seems impossible. The mind starts to rush about, thoughts come and go and you can think of everything but the object of your meditation. Do not be discouraged, for this is quite natural in the beginning. At this stage it is not the subject of your meditation that matters but the way you focus your mind upon it. Choose a simple object, such as a tree, an apple, a cloud, and try to hold it in your mind for several minutes as steady as you can. Try to concentrate all your thoughts upon it. Try to stop the mind wandering about, to switch off all thoughts of housework, dinner, cost of living. Concentrate as hard as you can, for you are aiming at thought control, one of the most difficult things for the average person to achieve. It is amazing how this simple exercise will develop the power of concentration.

It stands to reason that if you can control your mind you can develop a happier attitude to life. Try to defeat negative and destructive thoughts and your whole outlook and personality will improve, and in becoming master of yourself you will increase your influence on other people, for magnetism and vitality are infectious and attract others like the sun. You have only to think of the number of books and articles constantly appearing on the power of positive thinking to realise that there is something in the idea.

Some mental exercises and meditation themes suitable for western students are given below. They are all practised in the cross-legged position, with eyes closed, steady breathing established and mind calm and receptive.

1. *Gathering of the light*

This is the traditional preliminary to meditation. Everyone knows the meaning of inner enlightenment; in this exercise, by the uses of will-power, you are bringing about this illumination. Having established your rhythmical breathing, concentrate upon attaining stillness of mind. Let the thoughts come and go, trying to disregard them. Eventually, if you persevere, they will come less and less and one day you will find you have actually reached your goal, and the complete stillness that precedes enlightenment will be yours.

2. *Inversion of the mind's eye*

This could be your first exercise in meditation. It is a typical essay at self-analysis, an honest attempt to know yourself. Turn your thoughts in upon yourself, reviewing all your faults and weaknesses, admitting them and assessing them.

From inversion of the mind's eye, and acknowledgement of your failings, you proceed to the next two exercises, in which positive action is taken against the negative qualities you have revealed.

3. *I am stronger than fear*

Overcoming fear, conscious and unconscious, physical and moral, is one of the first steps in developing strength of character and serenity.

List all your fears . . . mental and physical . . . loss of material possessions, loss of friends, of health, of worldly position, etc. Try to think about them constructively, overcoming and rising above them. . . . For example, 'Even if I did lose my money or property it would not really be such a catastrophe; I would still retain my inner self, which no one can take from me.' And on the subject of physical fear. . . . 'I know that fear in time of emergency is destructive. It robs nine out of ten people of physical and mental faculties most needed at such a moment. I will not let this happen to me. It may never happen to me but I am preparing myself now in case it does.'

4. *I am master of myself*

Trying to exclude all other thoughts, take one by one the weaknesses or failings revealed by your self-analysis and systematically try to overcome them. Even for the best of us this could be a fairly long job, but persevere, concentrating on one at a time. Hesitation, procrastination, envy, jealousy, greed, inability to resist temptation, all should be rooted out, even if it takes you the rest of your life. Try to turn all these negative qualities into such positive ones as courage, strength and self-control and consequently you will achieve serenity.

There are four other suggested mental exercises which bring complete relaxation of the nervous system and which develop the powers of concentration and imagination. These are:

5. *Creating of a flower.* (This exercise and number 7 can be done sitting cross-legged or lying down in Position of Complete Rest.)

Choose your favourite flower and try to visualise it as clearly as you can. The mental image should be so strong that you feel you are actually creating it with the power of the imagination. Try to not only see it vividly but, as you breathe in and out, to smell its scent. If successful you will find that the exercise leads to complete relaxation of mind. Yoga believes that concentration on beautiful things helps to attain inner tranquillity.

6. *Mind mirror*

In this exercise, instead of choosing an external object, try to visualise your own self, as clearly as possible, seeing every detail as though in a looking-glass. Then try to project this image of yourself into the future, unchanged. This technique, a mild form of self-hypnosis, is an important exercise in delaying old age and is described in Chapter 3.

7. *Floating on a cloud*

Lying flat on the back, or sitting cross-legged, try to lose the sensation of your physical body, concentrating on the thought that with each exhalation you are growing lighter and lighter, as though really defying gravity forces. It is said that the ancient sages were able to actually raise themselves into the air by this exercise and were seen by their disciples floating as though on a cloud. It is not suggested that western students should expect to emulate them, but practice of the exercise is very beneficial to the nervous system.

8. *Protective cocoon*

Sitting cross-legged, inhale and exhale, directing *prana* through the millions of hair pores of the body and imagining that you are actually forming a kind of protective cocoon enclosing yourself from head to foot. Intense concentration is necessary, but if successfully practised the exercise leads to the subduing of all external influences, such as sound, light, heat or cold, leaving the practitioner entirely and completely alone with himself.

9. Finally, the exercise for transmuting sex energy could be practised if required (see Chapter 4).

Try to cultivate an optimistic but wise attitude to life and try to believe that everything is going to improve, not get worse. Try to give up fretting for what you cannot have and regretting what you did not do. Stop being negative and make up your mind to help yourself. It is not easy but the end is worth while working for. Patient practice of mental techniques, combined with toning-up *asanas* and regular relaxation, will help unhappy, restless women to achieve strength, serenity and inner peace.

7

Rest and relaxation

Several years ago an American magazine published a photograph showing a number of people waiting to cross the road at a New York traffic intersection. It was a fine summer morning and there were many young people in the crowd, yet every face showed unmistakable signs of tension, strain, anxiety or impatience.

This photograph comments more graphically than words on the effect of modern life on city-dwellers. Nine out of ten people, consciously or unconsciously, suffer from strain and tension, cannot find time to rest and, when they do, do not know how to relax. Nervous complaints, depression, insomnia, headaches, are common ailments; constipation, indigestion, ulcers and heart conditions ruin many lives. People go about with stomach nerves tensed up, with faces contracted and frowning; even in repose their hands are clenched; and when they go to bed they lie in screwed-up attitudes and wonder why they cannot sleep. Others who do manage to sleep complain that they wake as tired as they were before.

A woman who does not know how to relax will not retain her looks very long; even in youth her appearance can be spoilt by a tense and anxious expression, by tight-clenched fists or restlessly moving hands or feet; and one who cannot sit still, who speaks in shrill or strident tones is unattractive, no matter how fine her features or beautiful her figure.

Relaxation. Nervous tension

Relaxation should not be confused with 'having a rest'. One is a conscious and deliberate process while the other is more often than not a rather haphazard affair with varying results. You can lie down and have a rest for several hours and get up quite unrefreshed, but if you really know how to relax you can completely re-charge yourself in a matter of minutes.

The art of conscious relaxation, unknown to most western city-dwellers, is one of yoga's greatest gifts to us, but it is not a free gift. It must be worked for if it is to give its full benefits. Directions for practising this exercise—for it is an exercise—are given on page 117, and if you are suffering from nervous tension or similar conditions you should practise it as often as you can. Even normal healthy people should try to find time each day for at least a few minutes of *Savasana,* or Position of Complete Rest.

Sleep

Yoga has certain traditional beliefs about sleep, an important one being that it is not the number of hours of sleep but the quality of the sleep itself that counts; and that by improving this quality greater refreshment can be obtained in a shorter time. A knowledge of this fact has enabled many famous people to lead strenuous and demanding lives with a minimum of rest.

Yogi also believes that the position of the bed has an effect on sleep; that the human body, being a magnetic field, should be placed in opposition to the magnetic current of the earth. If it is, as for instance when the body lies in an east-west position, sleep may be restless and uneasy, particularly in the case of sensitive people. To avoid this disturbance it is suggested that the bed be placed with the head to the north and the feet to the south.

Insomnia is often allied to indigestion, caused by eating large meals too close to bedtime. If the body is too tired to digest a heavy evening meal there will usually be restless, fitful sleep or exhausting nightmares. If possible the main meal should be eaten at midday, and a lighter one in the evening; but if this is impossible time should be allowed for dinner to be digested before bed. In some southern European countries, where dinner is large and late, people stay up till all hours, talking and promenading, taking their rest during the day in the siesta, but this custom does not suit other parts of the world and individuals must try to adapt their habits to their own needs. In the same way they should note the effect of tea, coffee or other stimulants taken before bed, and if they are found to encourage insomnia they should be avoided at that time.

The bedroom should be well ventilated but not draughty, and as quiet and dark as possible; if noise and light cannot be eliminated put cotton wool in your ears and cover your eyes with a soft scarf. Even when the eyes are closed they are very susceptible to light.

A mattress that is too well sprung can be as disturbing as an uncomfortable one. Inner-spring mattresses are much more restful if they are put on a wooden platform.

Bedclothes should be warm but not heavy in weight, for if the body is supporting a load all night you will wake up feeling tired; and pillows should not be high, unless for some special reason such as asthma, heart trouble, etc.

One of the things that causes insomnia is staying up just a few minutes too long. No matter what the time is, everybody knows when they have reached the moment to go to bed, but unfortunately we often ignore this signal. We stay up, we go on working or talking or reading or watching television, and finally, when we do get into bed, the damage has been done. We have got a second wind, the mind is over-stimulated and we cannot get to sleep. We lie awake for hours, thinking, planning, tossing and turning, and the night is gone before we can recover the sleepiness we allowed to escape. Sleep in the early hours of the morning is never so refreshing as that which comes before midnight, for one is the sleep of exhaustion while the other is the sleep of refreshment.

Two things very beneficial to bad sleepers are deep breathing practised by an open window before getting into bed, or, if you live near the sea, a swim before bedtime. Sea-bathing is soothing and beneficial at any time, provided its effects are not cancelled out by lying too long in the hot sun, and at night it helps to relax the whole body before sleeping. Many people suffering from insomnia have also been helped by practice of the Triangular Pose described on page 133 (Pose of Tranquillity), which affects and soothes nervous centres in the back of the head; also by a rocking exercise which has much the same effect.

To perform this exercise, sit with the knees drawn up level with the shoulders, clasp the hands under the thighs and gently rock backwards as far as you can, trying to touch the floor over the head with the toes; then rock right forward until the head is down between the knees. Rock back and forth six or eight times, trying to keep a smooth and continuous movement; then lie down and relax.

Savasana is the best exercise to do before bed, either on the floor or when actually in bed. Train yourself to practise it properly and you will very likely be asleep before you have finished the fourth stage. If you are doing it in bed remove the pillow and lie perfectly flat.

Yoga suggests four different positions for restful sleep, each one associated with deep breathing.

Though you will not be able to retain the same position all night you will ensure proper respiration even in sleep if you have trained yourself to breathe in any of the four.

1. Lie flat on the back with the fingertips placed on the solar plexus. Inhale and exhale deeply and slowly, feeling the rise and fall of the abdomen. There is an almost hypnotic effect in this movement which induces drowsiness.

2. Lie flat on the stomach with the face turned to the left or right, and arms lying limply by the sides. You will have to remove your pillow to do this in comfort.

3. Lying on the left side, bend the left knee under you, with left arm stretched out under the head and right arm lying behind your back. Practise rhythmical abdominal breathing, pushing stomach out as you inhale and drawing it back with each exhalation.

4. The same as (3), lying on the right side.

Having done everything you can to ensure your rest, trying to eliminate or improve any external or physical causes of insomnia such as noise, light, uncomfortable beds, temperature, bedding or indigestion, turn your attention to your mental condition. It is unlikely that you will sleep well if your mind is eaten up with anxiety, bitterness, hatred or grief. Do the best you can with these enemies. Overcome those that you can control and try to dismiss those that you cannot.

Depression

Depression is a dangerous and insidious condition and women often find that having once given way to it they cannot shake it off. If there are no real circumstances to justify depression, or no physical causes such as disordered liver, anaemia or exhaustion following childbirth, it must be overcome by determination and persistence. There is nothing so guaranteed to lose your friends as a gloomy pessimistic attitude to life and no intelligent woman will let herself sink into this state. She will try to fight it by keeping herself occupied, by taking exercise and by proper relaxation to refresh her nervous system.

Since depression is often associated with lowered vitality, *asanas* which stimulate the thyroid should be practised, for this gland has a powerful effect on our vital energy and our whole attitude to life. Inverted poses as Shoulderstand (page 131) and Headstand (page 135) are two of the most important in this connection, also *Savasana* should be done as often as possible and such stimulating poses as Bird (page 146), Raven (page 147) and Spinal Twist (page 141).

The mental exercise on page 101 and 102, 'Inversion of the mind's eye', and 'I am master of myself', in which self-analysis is carried out, are important in trying to defeat depression and a negative attitude to life.

The case of a pupil, Mrs. C., should be an encouragement to women who feel the need of help in this matter. This woman, who was advised by her doctor to take up yoga, was forty-eight years of age. She had had her thyroid gland removed, was many stones overweight and looked twenty years older than her age. She suffered from persistent and overwhelming depression and nervous tension.

When she first came to the class she was so heavy and stiff that she literally could not raise her feet from the ground to get into the Shoulderstand and even when lifted by someone else into the upright position she was unable to retain it. She could not bend or stoop; she had no sense of balance. At first glance she might have appeared a hopeless proposition, but she had immense courage and determination and set herself to overcome her handicaps, practising religiously every day until her muscles began to loosen up. She propped herself up into the inverted poses against a table or wall until she could support herself. She went on a diet. She lost all her extra weight, and at the end of four months of yoga, having only one lesson a week, she was able to perform inverted, stretching and bending *asanas,* had trained herself to lock her legs in the Lotus Position and to stand on her head unaided. This remarkable woman, who incidentally had also lost an eye some time before in an accident, says that yoga has completely changed her life and her whole outlook. She is now a busy, cheerful and popular figure in her community.

PART TWO

Exercises and *Asanas*

If you have read the first part of this book you will know that yoga is not just a matter of doing exercises and tying yourself into knots, and that to really derive benefits the mind and character must be equally involved. This fact should be remembered while practising the *asanas* or bodily positions described in this section.

Do not be discouraged if you find some of the positions difficult or even apparently impossible to do. Most of them can be mastered by concentrated practice and in cases where they cannot, substitute others in their place. It is good to master the *asanas,* but what is even more important is the attempt and the practice, which is where the character and mind are brought into play, and which is one of the ways in which yoga differs from other systems of physical culture.

Never force or strain the body and never be deterred from trying by fear of failure or of appearing ridiculous. It must be admitted that in this respect women are much more realistic than men and much less self-conscious. Many women who begin by saying they could not do yoga because they look terrible in shorts or leotards quickly forget all about their appearance once they become interested in what they are doing. Most women are prepared to try anything that will help them attain an objective, particularly if the objective is the improvement of their looks, and we have seen women of all ages persevering to master difficult *asanas,* often overcoming considerable physical handicaps in the process.

We have selected thirty-one of the eighty-four traditional yoga *asanas,* all chosen for their importance to women. We have also included exercises for beautifying different parts of the body. Some of these exercises come from a series known as *The Magic of Slow Movements,* a practice not widely known in the west, which is somewhat similar to the ancient Chinese gymnastic of shadow boxing. They are body-building and body-moulding techniques of immense power, and must be practised very slowly, using the fullest constructive powers of the mind. They should be done before a mirror, or with the eyes closed and the mind's eye clearly visualising the muscles you are working on, and defining the result you are hoping to achieve . . . your body moulded into the shape you would like it to be.

An important thing to remember when doing the exercises or *asanas* is that everything you do in yoga has a purpose and is done for a reason. There is not a single gesture that has not been carefully thought out and included for its particular effect on a muscle, a gland, a nerve centre.

Sometimes variations of the same exercise may seem to be almost identical but you will find that there is some slight difference in the position of a foot or leg which changes the effect, putting pressure in a different place. An understanding of what you are doing will help you to practise with greater benefit and enjoyment.

8

Relaxation and limbering-up

Position of Complete Rest (Savasana)
Savasana, the yoga technique of relaxation, is an exercise made up of four stages, and is performed lying flat on the back, on the floor or some hard surface, with arms by the sides and eyes closed (Plate 2). Advanced students leave their eyes open, but the average practitioner needs to shut out light and distracting surroundings.

1. Start to consciously relax the muscles of the body, from the tips of the toes upwards, relaxing feet, ankles, calves, knees, thighs, abdominal muscles, chest and shoulders, arms and hands, facial muscles. Roll the eyes up under the closed lids; let the lower jaw go slack; try to relax the tongue in the mouth and wipe out any tension in the forehead, any tendency to frown. Every single muscle should be relaxed and the whole body limp and lifeless. After a few minutes pass your mind over your body to check that there are no points of tension, for instance the small of the back is sometimes overlooked and is a difficult part to relax at will, and if you find some muscles still re-

sisting try to induce them to give way, gradually persuading them, for forcing will only set up a resistance and tension.

2. With muscles relaxed, try to relax the nervous system, the feeling of inner tension. This is called Withdrawal of Nervous Energy and is more difficult to achieve than muscular relaxation. You may find it helpful to think of it as an actual withdrawal, like a tide going out; the ebbing away of all impulses from the nervous channels of the body, leaving them empty and limp. Induce a feeling of letting go, that nothing matters, and give yourself over to the idea that your body is becoming more and more leaden and lifeless, that you cannot even raise your hand, that you are sinking down, right through the floor.

3. Start deep and rhythmical breathing, practising full yoga breath (see page 124), pushing the stomach out as you inhale and drawing it back as you exhale. With each inhalation believe that you are inhaling *prana* with the air, and as you exhale you are breathing out only the air, retaining the *prana* in your body and sending it all through the system. In your rhythmical breathing you are doing two things: by inhaling *prana* you are re-charging your body, just as an exhausted battery is re-charged from the mains, and by slowing down the rate of breathing you are slowing down the tempo of the whole body and helping yourself to relax. Breath is thus a revitaliser and tranquilliser.

4. Now send your mind right away from your sur-

roundings, trying to detach yourself completely from your daily life, cares and responsibilities. Escape everything and try to transport yourself to some beautiful and peaceful place where life is just as you would like it to be. Yoga calls this Small Exit from the Physical Body, and you should try to make it a real exit or escape, to be more in this imaginary place you have chosen than in your actual surroundings. Finally, switch off all thoughts or pictures and try to keep your mind blank for a few seconds. This is the hardest thing of all to do and cannot be achieved at once. It will perhaps be a help if you roll your eyes up under the closed lids. Success with this part of the exercise leads to complete rest and relaxation of the mind. Then stretch your arms, yawn and open your eyes.

Savasana, which is also known as Pose of a Dead Man, when properly practised not only relaxes every muscle but every nerve and the mind itself. Traditionally it is done at the beginning and end of a yoga lesson, but it can be practised at any time, by anybody of any age. A few minutes of this exercise, properly done, is as refreshing as several hours of sleep, but if possible try to spend more than a few minutes on it. Older people will find longer periods very beneficial and everyone will profit from regular practice, particularly in cases of tension, insomnia, nervous disorders, high blood-pressure or heart conditions.

Limbering-up

Before beginning breathing cycles or *asanas* the body should be warmed-up by a few exercises designed to loosen the muscles, as dancers warm-up before practising.

1. With the body limp and relaxed, rotate each shoulder separately, concentrating on exercising the spine

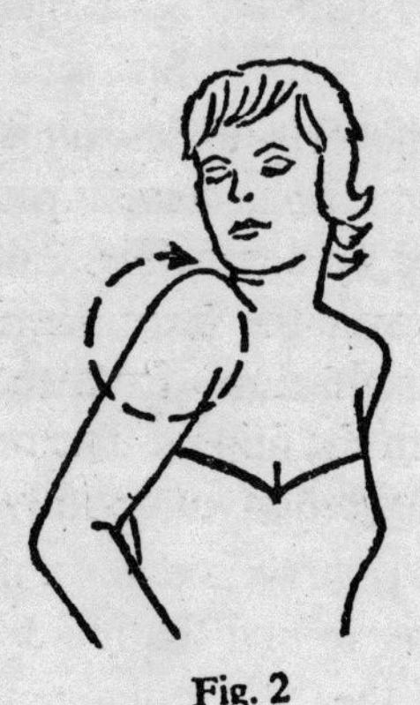

Fig. 2

(Fig. 2). First the movement is forward, like the action in swimming overarm; then, after half a dozen movements on each side, reverse the action so that it resembles a backstroke movement. You could then move both shoulders forward together, in a hunching-up circular movement and finally both back together, in exact reverse action, squeezing the spine between the shoulder-blades as they come back.

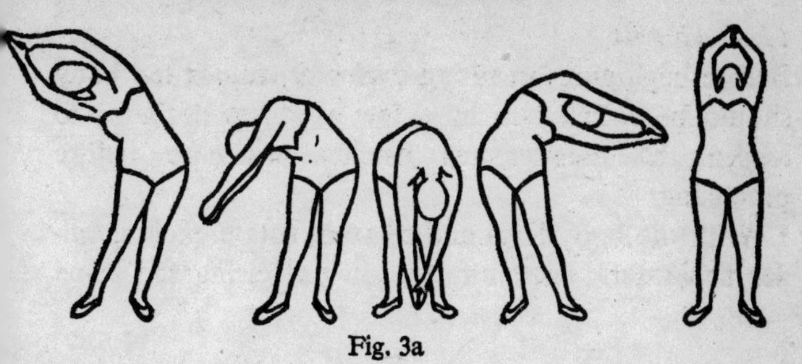

Fig. 3a

2. Combine the limbering-up movements into one loose rolling, circular action—arms up over the head, to the side, down and up again (Fig. 3a).
3. Stretch the arms over the head, then let the body fall limply forward, right down from the waist, trying to touch the floor with the fingers. The movement must be limp, with no suggestion of rigidity or resistance (Fig. 3b).

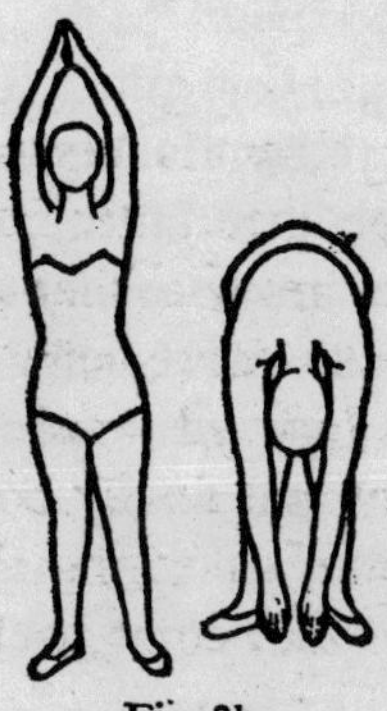

Fig. 3b

9

Breathing exercises

We have explained that the system of hatha yoga is based on breathing, that one of its main objectives is the achievement of breath control, and that yogis believe through such mastery man could eventually learn to control life itself. This is done through controlling the *prana* or Life Force which yoga teaches is in the air we breathe.

The pranic theory must be accepted by any student who really wishes to make progress, for it is a fundamental part of yoga philosophy. The higher forms of training are all devoted to the control of breath and advanced students spend more time in *pranayama* techniques — breath-control techniques — than in physical exercises. Most intelligent people can accept the theory and believe in the existence of *prana*, realising that there are so many things still unknown to man, and to those who remain sceptical it might be pointed out that fifty years ago anyone who talked about vitamins in food would have been regarded as extremely suspect.

According to yoga teaching, *prana* can be stored in

the body and then directed by the mind to different parts, with revitalising effects. A really advanced yogi can live on *prana* instead of food, for he knows how to replenish the cells of his body through his breathing. For most people, however, the most that will be achieved is a heightened feeling of well-being and an improvement in health and vitality, which, after all, are not inconsiderable achievements.

The seat of vital energy in the body is the solar plexus, and this is the storage place of *prana*. There are many breathing exercises which direct *prana* to this centre and others which send it to different parts of the body . . . the glands, vital organs, nervous plexuses, with re-charging and revitalising effects. Nothing can be done without the co-operation of the mind and will-power. In most cases the breathing exercises themselves are very easy to perform. The really difficult part is to control the mind and train it to work with and for you.

The yogic breath is a complete breath in which every part of the lungs is filled with air, increasing the intake of oxygen, and thus at the same time of *prana*. As you inhale you push out the stomach; this movement causes the diaphragm to descend and the lower part of the lungs to be filled. Then the middle part is filled by expanding the chest and finally the top of the lungs, by lifting and expanding the upper ribs. This is all done in one smooth, continuous movement, without any jerking.

As you exhale the stomach is drawn in, which lifts

the diaphragm, the ribs return to normal position and the air is expelled from the lungs. With the picture of this procedure in the mind's eye it is easy to understand why the use of the abdomen is so important in yoga breathing.

Put your hands on the abdomen, with fingertips touching, and practise rhythmical breathing. Inhale through the nose, counting six, then exhale counting six. This slow rhythm of about five breaths to the minute, instead of the usual fifteen to twenty, is the yoga tempo of deep breathing. As you inhale and exhale you will notice how your fingertips move apart and come together again, demonstrating the expansion and contraction of the stomach. You will remember from the chapter on relaxation and limbering-up that slowing down the breath is a method of helping the body to relax.

Cycle of breathing exercises for invigorating the system.

In all these exercises the breath is retained and then exhaled with the mind concentrated on the solar plexus and the mental image of *prana* being directed there.

1. Stand erect.
   Inhale full breath. Retain as long as comfortable. Exhale, forming mental image of *prana* directed to solar plexus.

2. Inhale.
   Raise arms forward, parallel with the floor.
   Grasp imaginary stick, retaining breath.
   Exhale and lower arms.

3. Inhale.
   Retain breath, tensing every muscle of the body.
   Exhale and relax.

4. Inhale.
   Rise up on tips of toes. Retain breath as long as you comfortably can.
   Exhale. Return to normal standing position.

5. Inhale.
   Raise both arms above head, putting palms together. Retain breath.
   Exhale. Lower arms.

6. Inhale.
   Press palms in front of chest in attitude of prayer.
   Retain breath.
   Exhale, releasing pressure and lowering arms.

7. Inhale. Retain breath.
   Combine the two previous movements. Raise arms above head, palms together, then slowly lower them—still pressed—until they are in attitude of prayer level with chest. Exhale.

8. *Ha Breath or Cleansing Breath*

   Stand with legs apart.

   Inhale deeply, raising the arms from the sides until they are stretched above the head.

   Throw the upper half of the body forward, bending from the waist, at the same time letting the arms fall forward and expelling the breath in a strong blast, making the sound HA. Let the body hang limply from the waist, arms swinging, head hanging loosely as you repeat the HA sound several times.

   Stand up and repeat the inhaling and exhaling twice more.

This Ha or Cleansing Breath is designed to completely fill the lungs with fresh air and completely expel all tired or stale air that is lying in them. It should be practised three times at the end of every breathing cycle and is an important means of refreshing and re-charging the body at any time when tiredness is felt.

Further breathing exercises

9. Inhale full breath.

   Raise arms forward. Retain breath, and, clenching fists, pull arms back until hands are level with shoulders. Extend arms again, pull back again. Drop arms to sides and exhale through mouth.

10. Inhale.
    Locking the breath, raise arms forward in a circular swinging movement, crossing them in the front and continuing the swing in a complete circle, twice; then at the end of the second circle change direction and reverse swing, *e.g.* At first the arms are swung forward and upwards in a circular movement then forwards and *downwards.*
    Drop arms to sides and exhale through mouth.

11. Inhale slowly.
    Retain breath, tapping the chest at top of lungs.
    Turn head to one side and exhale through mouth in a series of short sharp breaths.

12. Inhale slowly.
    Retain breath, massaging the lower ribs.
    Turn head to side and exhale through pursed-up lips, in long continuous breath.
    Conclude cycle with another cleansing breath.

If possible, devote three to five minutes every day to breathing exercises. To be effective, at least sixty deep breaths should be performed during the day. The best time of all is early morning on getting up, but if you suffer from insomnia you will find it helpful to also do deep breathing by an open window before going to bed.

10

Asanas

SITTING POSES

The best-known sitting positions in yoga are the cross-legged . . . Simple, or Easy Pose, Pose of an Adept, Half-Lotus, Lotus or Buddha Pose and the Free Pose. All are described here, with the addition of another sitting position known as Pose of a Hero.

The cross-legged positions are the traditional yoga positions for the practice of meditation and are also used for breathing exercises and techniques designed to increase mental powers. In these positions, especially in the Lotus, the blood circulation is slowed down in the legs and increased in the top of the body, including the head, so that thinking becomes easier and clearer. The back and neck are kept in one straight line and the hands rest on the knees in a relaxed manner. The hands may also be loosely clasped together, or placed one upon the other, close to the body, with palms upwards, the back of the right hand in the palm of the left.

Most women find the Lotus position very difficult, though there are a few who, due to the way the legs are set on the hips, can perform it immediately. These women usually have long slender legs, with slim thighs. Women with short legs or heavy thighs have considerable trouble, and some never achieve the position. These people should use the Half-Lotus, or Pose of an Adept, or the Easy Pose. Others, though finding it hard at first, can eventually master the full Lotus after a good deal of practice and perseverance.

1. *Easy Pose.* Sit with the legs crossed, hands resting on knees, and back and neck in one straight line (Plate 3).

2. *Pose of an Adept.* Sit with left foot close to the body and the right foot placed between the left calf and thigh. Plate 5 must be studied carefully, for verbal directions are not easy to follow. The legs can be changed, bringing the right foot close to the body and placing the left foot between right thigh and calf.

3. *Half-Lotus.* Sit in the Pose of an Adept, as above, but instead of putting the right foot between calf and thigh, bring it up higher, close to the groin, where it will effect pressure on one of the main arteries of the body (see Plate 7). Right and left leg can be used alternately.

4. *Lotus or Buddha position.* In this pose both legs are interlocked, with the heels effecting pressure on

the main arteries near the groins. This increased pressure gradually slows down the circulation in the legs and directs the blood supply to the upper part of the body and head, stimulating and clarifying the process of thought (see Plate 8).

5. *Free Pose.* The legs are not crossed in the ordinary way but placed one before the other, with knees as close as possible to the floor (see Plate 6). Starting, for instance, with the left leg, bring the heel close to the body as though about to perform Pose of an Adept, or Half Lotus; then place right heel in front of and almost in line with the left heel. This automatically spreads the knees wide apart and they can be gently encouraged to lie flatter on the floor by pressure of the hands.

6. *Pose of a Hero.* This position is usually associated with a mental exercise concerned with the development of inner strength, and the illustration (Plate 4) should be studied carefully for the position of the legs. It is practised on alternate sides. Starting with right leg, bend the knee and bring the leg to the side of the body, so that the knee points forward and the foot is to the back. Then raise the left foot and rest it in the Half-Lotus position on the right thigh. Hold the pose, practising rhythmical breathing and with the mind concentrated on the thought of developing inner strength and courage; then change legs and continue concentration. This position is said to have been

taught to Alexander the Great by the yogis during his invasion of India.

Apart from their importance as meditation poses, the cross-legged *asanas* have certain physical effects on the body. They are all important exercises in antenatal training and mastery of the Lotus is said to facilitate painless childbirth. Lotus Pose is also recommended for certain internal female disorders (see table on pages 187–9) and for helping to develop poise, confidence and tranquillity.

INVERTED POSES

The inverted poses are an extremely important part of yoga training, for their effects on the body are vital and widespread. The five poses described here can, between them, restore youthfulness, delay ageing, prevent wrinkles, cure insomnia and nervous conditions, and improve mental powers. These results are brought about by interference with the blood circulation, by sending a supply of extra blood to glands and nervous centres and by putting pressure on certain glands. The inverted poses also counteract the pull of central gravity forces which cause sagging tissues and the displacement of vital organs.

Shoulderstand. Also known as Candle Pose (Plate 9). Lie down on the back and slowly lift the legs and body up into a vertical position, supporting yourself by placing the hands in the region of the shoulder-blades, taking the weight on the elbows and upper arms. The body should eventually be in one straight line from the shoulders. Chin must be pressed tightly to chest.

Close the eyes, breathe deeply and concentrate on the thought of rejuvenation, and on what this pose is actually doing to your body. The blood drained from the raised legs is flowing into the rest of the body, stimulating and feeding it, and through the action of the chin pressed to the chest it is held in the region of the thyroid and parathyroid glands which thus receive the maximum benefit. Due to the influence of these glands on the rest of the endocrinal system, every other gland in the body is also toned-up and benefited. The effects of ageing, failure of mental and sexual powers, excess weight and loss of vitality are all improved by this remarkable pose, which is one of the most important *asanas* in hatha yoga.

In the beginning hold the position for only a short time—a couple of minutes—but as you become stronger you should hold it for as long as possible. The longer you can retain it, the greater will be the benefits. If you are not strong enough to hold it alone at first support your legs against a wall or heavy table.

When you are ready to come down slowly lower the legs over the head, placing hands flat on the floor and keeping the knees straight and legs stiff, and try to touch the floor with your toes. This is the *Plough Pose* (page 139) (Plate 16). Retain for a minute or so, concentrating the mind on the spinal column and on the thought that the roots of the spinal nerves are being toned-up and fed with an extra supply of arterial blood. Rhythmically breathe in and out while holding the pose. Then come down and completely relax.

In all the following inverted poses deep breathing should be practised while the position is held.

Half-Shoulderstand or Half-Candle (Plate 10)

This position is very similar to the previous one, but instead of supporting the back with the hands, the hips are held, with the body at an angle of about 30 degrees from the vertical, and the extra supply of blood is drawn to the skin of the face, nourishing each cell of the facial tissues. Breathe rhythmically through the nose.

Half-shoulderstand is known as one which prevents and destroys wrinkles and helps to retain a youthful appearance for many years. To get the best results it should be practised regularly, at first holding it for about a minute, then increasing to five minutes or more. Never hold longer than is comfortable.

To conclude, bring the legs slowly down over the head, slightly bending the knees so that you can take hold of the toes. Pull the legs out straight with a slight jerk, try to touch the floor above the head with the toes, then release them and slowly lower the legs and arms to the floor. Relax completely, with arms by the sides.

Triangular Pose or Pose of Tranquillity

Lie on the back and stretch the arms on the floor above the head. Keeping the knees straight, raise the legs to form an angle of 45 degrees with the body (Plate 11). Raise the arms and rest the knees on the palms of the hands. The elbows must be kept stiff and the weight of the legs literally resting on the hands, with pressure on the back of the neck. If you let your elbows bend, the weight of the legs will pull you over. This is a balancing pose and it may be necessary to experiment until the right position is found for the hands, for everyone's arms and legs are a different length and the position will vary accordingly.

To finish this pose bring the legs down over the head; split the knees apart; take hold of your knees and press them to the ground on each side of the head (Plate 13). This is called Choking Position. It is a variation of the Plough Pose, and puts pressure on the thyroid gland. Finally, lower legs and arms slowly to the floor and relax. This *asana* has great power to calm the nerves and induce peaceful sleep by increasing blood circulation in nerve centres at the back of the neck and head.

Balancing Shoulderstand

Lying on the back with arms stretched above head, as in Triangular Pose, slowly raise the legs and body into the air until they form a vertical line from the shoulders. When the balance is established slightly incline the legs towards the head and slowly raise both arms upwards. Hold the pose for two or three minutes, breathing rhythmically, then bring the legs down over the head in the Choking Pose described above, and, after pressing the knees to the floor, lower arms and legs and relax.

Balancing Shoulderstand, like all inverted poses, is a rejuvenator and is said to increase and improve mental powers through directing extra blood to the brain. The pineal gland at the back of the head is also stimulated and yogis believe that this can lead to development of higher faculties, such as telepathy and clairvoyance.

Head Pose or Headstand

Kneel down on a rug or carpet, making sure it will not slip about, and rest your forearms on the floor. The fingers should be interlaced and the hands resting on the outer edges of the palms, forming a little fence. Lean forward and put your head into this little enclosure (Fig. 4). Straighten your legs and begin to walk in towards your body. When you can get no

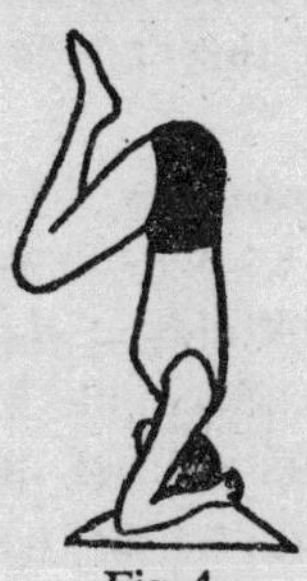

Fig. 4

closer try to lift your legs from the ground into a bent position. (At first it may be necessary to kick up, but when the muscles of the back are stronger they should be raised gradually.) Then slowly straighten out the legs until the whole body is in a straight line (Plate 14). Elbows and forearms should be kept parallel and fairly close together, since they are holding the weight of the body, and back should not be arched, for this will affect balance. Deeply inhale and exhale.

To come down, slowly bring the knees in towards the stomach, in a folding-up movement; then gradually lower the torso until the feet are on the ground.

In the beginning you should never try to do Headstand alone, and if you have no one to help you, practise against a wall to prevent any danger of falling. Do not try to hold the position for more than a few seconds at first. This time can be increased with experience but should never be too long. The object of the deep breathing practised during the Headstand is to ensure a good supply of oxygen for the extra blood that is being sent to the head. The Headstand is usually practised at the end of a lesson, after rest and relaxation.

The Headstand is probably the most famous of all yoga *asanas* and best-known to westerners, who have seen pictures of well-known public figures standing on their heads and read about the benefits it is said to bring. These benefits are not imaginary and are so widespread that this *asana* is known as the King of Yoga Positions. It is a great rejuvenator and restorer of lost vitality and sex-powers; it tones up the whole body through its effects on glands, nervous centres and on the brain itself. The extra arterial blood sent to the head improves mental faculties . . . memory, concentration, clarity of thought . . . and benefits nose, throat, ears and eyes; and the reversed position of the body acts as a counter-measure against central gravity forces (see Chapter 3—Delaying old age). Such diverse conditions as prolapsed uterus, varicose veins and asthma are said to be improved.

For normal people there is no prohibition against practising Headstand, but in certain cases it is definitely forbidden. Women with high blood-pressure must not attempt it, nor should those with heart trouble. Those who are very much overweight and over fifty years of age should use great caution, stopping immediately there is any sign of trouble, and the same applies to women with weak eye capillaries (bloodshot eyes). The reader will have no difficulty in understanding why these prohibitions are made (since all conditions described forbid extra blood sent to the head) and use her own discretion or consult her doctor. For the rest, the Headstand can bring only unending benefit.

STRETCHING CYCLE

Yoga teaches that old age begins with stiffening of the backbone and joints, and to fight this stiffening cycles of stretching poses have been evolved. Though they are mainly designed to keep the spine supple they also have the same effect on the joints and if practised regularly will keep the whole body limber.

Even if some of the positions seem impossible to achieve at first you should persevere, because it is the attempt that is important, and with practice the muscles will soon loosen up and permit you to do the *asanas* easily and gracefully. The main thing to remember is that nothing should ever be forced.

Arch Gesture

Sitting with the back straight and the right leg stretched before you, bend the left knee and press the sole of the foot flat against the inside of the right thigh, forming a right-angle with the thighs (Plate 17). Inhale, and as you exhale, bend forward and take hold of the right foot. Try to touch the right knee with your forehead. Hold for a couple of seconds, then sit up, change legs and repeat.

In this exercise, and in all the others of the stretching cycle, draw in the stomach as you bend forward. The forward movement massages the abdominal organs, the position of the legs in the different variations effecting pressure in different places.

Variation of Arch Gesture (Plate 19)

Sitting in the same position, with right leg stretched, bend the left knee as before but this time place the foot up on the right thigh, close to the body, in the Half-Lotus position. Try to keep the knee flat on the floor, if necessary working on it with the hand, gently pressing it down.

Inhale, exhale and stretch forward as before, trying to touch the knee with the head. Then sit up, change legs and repeat.

In the beginning it is easier if you take hold of the ankle of the outstretched leg and pull yourself down a little. It is astonishing how quickly the body will respond to practice.

Head-to-knee Pose. Standing (Plate 22)

With feet together, inhale, and as you exhale, bend forward, keeping the knees stiff and sliding the hands down the outside of the legs until you can take hold of your ankles. Touch the knees with the forehead, then stand up and repeat the exercise.

This *asana* and the sitting version described below are important in their effect on the abdominal organs. They help to cure indigestion and constipation when practised in moderation. They also tone up liver, kidneys and pancreas and improve menstrual disorders. They reduce fat and are said to increase height.

In the *Sitting Pose* both legs are outstretched, and after inhalation the breath is exhaled as you bend forward. Take hold of the toes and pull the body down until the head rests on the knees. The elbows should be resting on the ground on each side of the legs. Hold for a few seconds, then repeat (Plate 22).

Plough Pose (Plate 16)

This *asana* is usually practised with the Shoulder-stand, forming the second part of the exercise, but is really a separate position.

Lying on your back, bring your legs over the head and try to touch the floor with your toes. Arms remain flat on the floor, at sides. Hold it for a few seconds, deeply breathing in and out, then lower the legs, as in the Inverted Positions, and relax.

In a *Variation of the Plough* the arms are stretched above the head and the toes held, keeping the legs quite straight, while deep inhalation and exhalation is performed.

Apart from keeping the spine supple, the Plough is recommended for constipation and digestive troubles, for menstrual disorders and liver enlargement, and for reducing fat on the abdomen.

The Archer

Sit with the right leg outstretched. Step over it with the left, placing left foot flat on the floor beside the right knee (Plate 21). Put the left hand on the toes of the right foot; take hold of the left foot with the right hand. Inhale, exhale and slowly pull the left foot up towards the head, trying to touch the point between the eyebrows with the big toe. Lower the leg, change sides and repeat. The action is similar to that of an archer pulling back his bow to release an arrow, and the bent arm, the one that is doing the pulling, should be held up and out from the body. If the elbow is kept in and cramped it will be difficult to perform the exercise, apart from the ugliness of such a movement.

This *asana* will help to reduce fat on stomach and

hips, it will improve digestion and constipation, loosen the spine and generally 'pep-up' the body.

Sideways Swing

Sitting with both legs to the right (see Plate 25), raise the arms and loosely link them over the head. Inhale, exhale and swing the arms and body over the bent legs as you breathe out. Perform several times, then change legs to other side and repeat movement.

This exercise will reduce the waistline and give suppleness of the spine.

Yoga Spinal Twist

The easiest way to get into this position is to do it immediately after the Sideways Swing, while the legs are still bent to one side. Leaving the left leg in position on the floor, step over it with the right, keeping the thigh close to the body and with calf and thigh forming a triangle with the floor. Slightly turn the body until you can place the right knee under the left armpit, with the left arm extended to the right foot. The right arm is bent behind the back. Inhale, exhale and twist your body as far as you can to the right, trying to see directly behind you. Change to opposite arms and legs and repeat the twist. Study the illustration (Plate 20), which will explain more clearly than any words can do.

The Spinal Twist is a very stimulating *asana* and its effects are felt immediately in a sensation of increased vitality and well-being. It keeps the spine elastic, sends extra blood to the spinal nerves and massages and tones-up abdominal organs, relieving constipation and dyspepsia. It also reduces fat on stomach, hips and waistline.

Cobra (Plate 26)
Lie on the floor, face downwards, palms flat on the floor, level with the chest, and feet stretched out flat. Inhale and lift the head and neck upwards and backwards; then, by contracting the muscles in the back, raise the chest, exerting a powerful pressure on the small of the back. The body from the navel downwards should be pressed in the small of the back. Lower the body as you exhale, then repeat the exercise three times. In the first two upward movements the chin is raised, in the second two it is pressed to the chest.

Cobra is an important exercise for women, apart from its effect on the spine and adrenal glands. It helps to correct menstrual disorders and to tone-up the sex glands and reproductive organs. It also tones-up the other abdominal organs and relieves constipation.

This exercise, and the three described below, all stretch the spine in the opposite way to the Plough Pose, and for this reason are best practised after that *asana*.

The Bow (Plate 27)
Lying on the floor, as in Cobra Pose, bend your

knees so that you can take hold of your ankles. Inhale, raise the head and shoulders and at the same time pull on the ankles, forming the body into a bow. Hold for a few seconds, then relax. Repeat several times, with a smooth movement, not jerking.

This exercise firms the thighs, slims the abdomen and develops and firms the bust. It also stimulates the spinal nerves, peps-up the whole body and benefits the female reproductive system.

The Locust (Plate 30)

Lying face downward on the floor, bring the arms very close to the sides, or, in the early stages, under the thighs, with elbows straight and fists clenched. Turn the fists so that the knuckles are touching the floor, then with a quick movement raise both legs, keeping them close together and straight, and at the same time inhale deeply. Hold the breath and the pose for two or three seconds, then lower the legs slowly and exhale. Repeat two or three times.

Locust benefits women through its effect on the ovaries and uterus, helping to correct disorders in these organs. It also strengthens abdominal muscles and spine and improves the whole respiratory system.

Fish Pose (Plate 31)

If possible lock the legs in the Lotus position, otherwise cross them in the ordinary way. Lean back, lower the body to the floor, arching the spine and resting on the crown of the head. Hands should be resting on toes. Alternatively they could be crossed behind the neck, with the right hand under the left shoulder-blade and the left under the right shoulder-blade. Head is resting on the crossed arms. Deep breathing should be maintained in this pose, for the lungs are free of any restriction and can be completely filled and completely emptied. Fish Pose also benefits the reproductive organs, stimulates the ovaries and helps to correct menstrual troubles. It is an aid in overcoming constipation.

The Wheel (Plate 28)

The safest and easiest way to get into the Wheel position is to start lying on your back on the floor. Bring up the knees, with the feet flat on the floor and close to the body, and bend the arms so that the palms of the hands rest on each side of the head. The hands should be turned so that the fingers are pointing towards the feet (see Fig. 5).

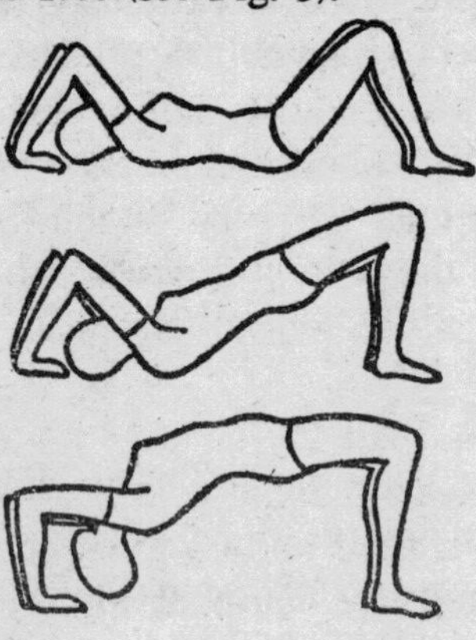

Fig. 5

Try to lift yourself up, keeping soles and palms flat on the floor, until the spine is completely arched and the body forms a semi-circle with the floor. At first you may be able to lift only the hips, finding the head and shoulders too heavy to raise, but with practice you will get stronger and the spine more supple. Young girls and children have no difficulty doing the Wheel and it is a very well-known acrobatic exercise, usually accompanied by spectacular variations.

Its importance as practised in yoga is to exercise and stimulate the spine and spinal nerves. It also benefits the female reproductive system and helps to correct constipation and digestive troubles. It prevents excess weight and is an excellent toning-up method.

It can also be practised from a standing position, bending backwards as far as possible, eventually until the hands are on the floor, palms flat and fingers turned towards feet. This is extremely difficult and dangerous and the first method of practice is the best for most people. Those who feel capable and confident enough to try from the standing position should have someone to hold the back in the beginning or to ease their way down by sliding the hands down a wall, which will help to control tendencies to fall.

Supine-Pelvic Pose (Plate 29)

Sit on your heels, as in Head of a Cow Pose (Plate 35). Then split your heels and try to sit between them, keeping knees together. Lean back and helping yourself by leaning first on your hands, then on your elbows, lower yourself to the floor, arching the back and resting on the crown of the head. Hands are held in front of body in position of prayer. Breathe rhythmically.

If you can do this in comfort you could then lower the body until the shoulders are flat on the floor, with arms stretched out above the head, or folded under the small of the back. A variation is to lean back without trying to sit between the heels, giving a higher arch to the back.

This *asana* helps to cure digestive troubles, constipation and disorders of the female reproductive system. It beautifies the neck, firms the thighs and strengthens the spine. It is said to help in sciatica and sexual debility.

RAISED POSITIONS

The practice of raised positions helps to maintain lightness and buoyancy, physical qualities which most people lose when their youth has gone. Yoga teaches that this is unnecessary, and that no one should lose their relative strength, the ability to lift their own weight. The raised poses were designed to counteract the tendency towards increasing heaviness with passing years.

Pose of a Bird

Squat on the floor with the knees apart. Put the hands on the floor, palms downwards, between the knees, and spread out the fingers like the claws of a bird. Pressing the inside of the knees against the outside of the arms, slowly lean forward until the feet are off the floor. Inhale as you rise, exhale as you come down. Try to perform the movement smoothly, not jumping or jerking, and keep the toes together, forming the bird's tail (Plate 32).

This *asana* is a pepping-up medium and helps to keep the body light and slim and the face free from wrinkles for the movement sends extra blood to the face and stimulates and feeds the tissues.

Pose of a Raven, Right and Left Aspects

This is a variation of the Bird Pose and is performed in the same way, with a difference in the position of the arms. Instead of being between the knees they are placed to the side . . . on the left for Left Aspect, on the right for Right Aspect. The knees are held close together.

Inhale, lean forward with the side of the bent knee pressed against the outside of the arm, and try to rise up, lifting the feet from the ground, and with the weight of the body balanced against the arm. If practising Right Aspect it will be the left leg pressed against the right arm (see Plate 33).

The benefits of this pose, which must be practised on both sides, are the same as those of the Bird.

ABDOMINAL CONTRACTIONS

The yoga abdominal contractions are considered to

be among the most important of all yoga exercises and are essential for anyone wishing to improve digestion and correct constipation. To get the best results they should be practised every day, always and *only* on an empty stomach, and preferably first thing in the morning, on getting up. The majority of people find that as they get older their whole eliminative system becomes more and more sluggish, until they are chronically constipated, and consequently in a permanent state of indifferent health. They are not really ill, but they are never completely well and are always complaining of headaches, depression and vague feelings of malaise. They are, in fact, suffering from slow poisoning caused by wastes and impurities left in the system and absorbed back into the bloodstream through the walls of the bowels. It is unlikely that they will actually die of constipation but they certainly cannot enjoy living while it exists.

Apart from the feeling of ill-health that it brings, constipation is now believed to be one of the chief causes of ageing in the human body, and this belief, which the yogis have held for thousands of years, is now being confirmed by scientists and researchers specialising in geriatrics (the study of senility).

For women, the abdominal contractions also have a special importance, for the movements of the internal organs affect and stimulate the sex glands, the uterus and the whole reproductive system. Menstrual disorders can be helped and ovarian deficiency, as well as sexual debility; but the contractions must never be practised during menstruation or during pregnancy. Some authorities also forbid them to young girls whose periods are not yet properly established and who are still going through puberty.

Uddiyana (Plate 37)

This exercise can be done sitting or standing. If in standing position place feet about eighteen inches apart, rest your hands on your thighs and slightly bend the knees. Lean forward a little with the weight on the hands. Inhale, completely exhale, then contract the abdominal muscles, drawing the stomach in as far as possible towards the spine, and at the same time raising the diaphragm. The abdomen should be quite hollow with a deep concavity under the ribs. Hold for a few seconds, then relax and repeat the process. All air must be expelled from the lungs before the contraction can be made. Chin is pressed to chest.

In the second stage of the exercise try to bring about a flapping movement of the abdomen by rapidly contracting and relaxing the muscles you are working on, in, out, in, out, several times. As you master the techniques, and your control improves, increase the number of contractions.

The same procedure is followed in the sitting position. It is performed sitting cross-legged, or preferably in Pose of an Adept or Lotus position.

Nauli

This is a more advanced form of the stomach contractions and is usually practised after *Uddiyana*. After contracting the stomach and raising the diaphragm to form the hollow in the abdomen, the abdominal recti muscles must be separated and exercised in a rotary movement. This is not only difficult to do but also difficult to explain and really needs personal demonstration. Study Plate 38 and try to realise what is being done. The abdominal recti muscles, which are rooted in the pit of the stomach, just above the pubic bone, are contracted, forming a hard column right up the centre of the abdomen. They are then contracted on the right side, then on the left, in each case making the same muscular column on the appropriate side of the body. When the actual contractions or separations are mastered they are performed quickly, one after another, centre, left, centre, right side, centre, left side, etc., in a continuous churning movement, which to an observer looks like one action but which is really a series of closely integrated contractions. If you have ever seen a Polynesian hula dancer you will have some idea of the movement, though in Nauli the hips are not rotated. Everything is confined to the abdominal muscles.

There is no doubt that this technique is hard for most people and that many never master it at all, but it is not impossible to achieve and is so beneficial that it is worth persevering with. Practise in front of a mirror so that you can watch what is happening, and remember that in first separating the central muscles into a column you should make a *forward* and *downward* thrusting movement in the pit of the stomach. Try also closing your eyes, picturing in your mind what you are trying to do and relaxing any tendency to force body or mind. In this state, watching yourself performing the exercise in your mind's eye, you can suddenly find that you are actually doing it.

BALANCING POSES

The balancing poses of yoga are not only designed to affect the body but also have a powerful effect on the mind and the inner-life. They give grace, balance and control, both physically and mentally, resulting in a feeling of peace and tranquillity.

Tree Pose

Standing on the left leg, lift the right foot and place it on the left thigh with the sole turned out. It should be as high up as possible with the heel near the groin. Raise the arms over the head and place palms together. Hold the pose for a couple of minutes, deeply breathing in and out, with the eyes focused on the tip of the nose. Relax, change legs and repeat (Plate 39).

A *variation of Tree Pose* is to stand on the left foot, holding the right foot behind you and with the left arm raised in line with the body (Plate 39). After holding for a minute or so, deeply breathing in and out, relax and change sides.

Increase the time of holding the pose until you can manage three or four minutes, standing quite steadily.

Eagle Pose

Stand upright, then slightly bend the left knee. Wind the right leg round it, as in Plate 40. Bend forward a little and wind the arms into the same position, resting the elbow of the underneath arm on the right thigh, and with the chin resting on the back of the hand. Eyes should be focused on the tip of the nose. Hold for a few seconds, then relax, change arms and legs and repeat.

This pose, which sounds complicated, should be partly familiar to most women, for it is a very common feminine practice to sit with the legs twisted round each other in exactly this position.

Eagle Pose strengthens knees and ankles and also helps in cases of sterility and sexual debility, for it puts direct pressure on the ovaries.

MISCELLANEOUS POSES

The following poses should be practised for the benefits described in each case:

Pose of a Cat (Plate 23)

Kneel down, lean forward and get into a kind of all-fours position, with the palms of the hands flat on the floor. Keep the arms straight and let the head hang down. Now start to manipulate the spine, keeping the rest of the body still. Let the spine take all the movement, depressing it down into a concave line, then raising it up into a hump, then down again, then up, just as a cat does when it is exercising its backbone. Do not let the elbows bend or the arms sag as you move, otherwise the effect will be lost.

Pose of a Cat is recommended for the spine and is also much used as an ante-natal and post-natal exercise (see Appendix I).

Head of a Cow Pose

Sit on your heels, or on your crossed ankles. Bend your arms so that you can grip your hands together behind your back, level with the shoulder-blades. For instance, the left arm will be bent upwards behind the back and the right arm bent down over the shoulder so that the hands can meet (Fig. 6).

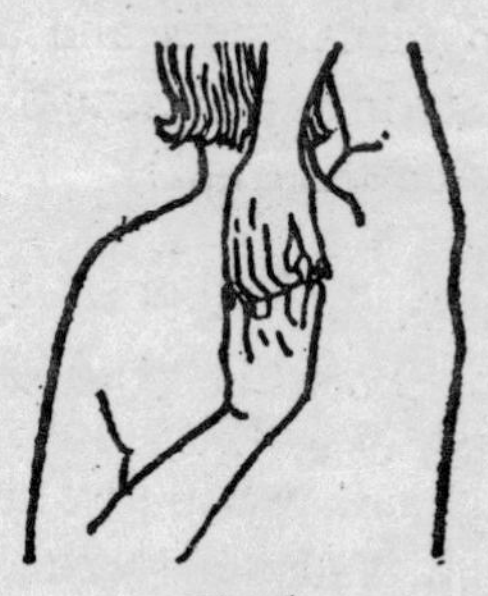

Fig. 6

Sit in this pose and inhale and exhale: then lean forward and touch the floor with the forehead, trying to stop the hands coming ungripped. Sit up, change sides and repeat.

Apart from benefiting arms, chest and back muscles, this pose and its forward movement is a beautifying exercise for the face, for extra blood is brought up to the head to feed the skin and tissues (Plate 35).

Yoga-mudra (Plate 34)

Sit in the Lotus position and clasp your hands behind your back. Inhale and bend forward until the forehead touches the floor. Hold the breath and the pose for a few seconds, then sit up, exhale and massage the face by tapping with fingertips.

Yoga-mudra benefits the abdominal and reproductive organs and is also a beautifier, in the same way as Head of a Cow, by sending extra blood to the face.

It may also be practised in the following way: Inhale, exhale as you lean forward and retain position for five seconds.

Pose of a Child

Sit on your heels, as in Head of a Cow. Lean forward and let the forehead rest on the floor with arms lying limply by the sides and trying not to rise up at the back. Inhale and exhale peacefully. Sit up and relax.

This pose, which is also a relaxation pose, is a rejuvenator and beautifier through its effect of bringing extra blood to the face (Plate 36).

Aswini-mudra

Sit comfortably in the cross-legged position, or sit on

your heels. Inhale, exhale and at the same time contract the muscles of the anus, drawing them in as though to prevent a bowel action. Hold the contraction for a few seconds, then relax, inhale again and repeat the exercise. The movement should be contraction while exhaling, relaxing while inhaling. Practise gradually at first, then try to do the contractions more rapidly, continuing for several minutes.

The contractions massage and tone-up the female sex organs, and if you concentrate on practice you will be able to exercise the vagina in the same way. *Aswini-mudra* is designed for both sexes, but since the muscular walls of rectum and vagina adjoin in the female body it is specially beneficial for women (see Chapter 4—Yoga and sex).

This *asana* is helpful in constipation and haemorrhoids and it also benefits nerves and organs of the reproductive system. It is thus an important exercise in the treatment of sexual debility. It is often included in ante- and post-natal exercises (see Appendix I—Yoga and natural childbirth).

Pose of a Camel

Kneel down and slightly separate the legs. Lean back, with the arms stretched out straight behind you, lowering yourself back until the hands can take hold of the heels. Keep the arms quite stiff and do not bend the elbows. Arch your back and let your head fall back loosely. Hold the pose (Plate 24), inhaling and exhaling, then come up and relax.

Pose of a Camel exercises the spine and tones-up the spinal nerves. It also beautifies the neck, discourages fat on waist and abdomen and benefits the female organs of reproduction.

11

Body-moulding and body-building techniques

In this chapter we have given a number of exercises and *asanas* which will improve and develop different parts of the body . . . bust, stomach, waistline, hips, legs, arms, back and shoulders. The slow movements described are taken from the series mentioned on page 113 and have been selected for their importance to women. Descriptions of the *asanas* will be found on the page-numbers given.

Remember that the slow movement must be done using fully the constructive power of the mind, and should be practised before a looking-glass or with the mind's eye concentrated on the muscles you are working on, trying to see yourself as you would like to be. As already mentioned, the mind and imagination play a most important part in the practice of all the slow movements.

Each movement should be done four times. Regular practice will give remarkable results, even in some cases where damage has already been done to the tissues by age, lack of exercise or loss of weight.

For firming and preserving the bust

1. *Pulling a rope.* Standing with feet together, raise the arms above the head and grasp an invisible rope. Pull down on it, tensing the muscles of the chest, then relaxing. Repeat four times, relaxing between each movement.

2. *Pressing down.* Raise the arms from the sides and with palms turned down, bring them forward in a semi-circular movement until they are stretched in front, parallel to each other; then continue the downward movement, pressing down with chest muscles tensed. When the arms are about level with the waist, on their downward journey, relax the tension, but keep the movement going . . . up again from the sides, forward, downwards in a continuous circling movement.

3. *Pressing in.* Move the arms out from the side, then bring them in together, tensing them, until the clenched fists meet in front of the stomach. Relax and repeat.

4. Perform the same movement but continue the inward movement of the arms until the fists cross in front of the stomach. Repeat.

5. In a further variation of the same exercise the arms are brought in from the sides, keeping the elbows held high, about level with the chest. The clenched fists should be brought together level with the middle of the chest. Repeat.

Although these exercises may appear very similar, the slight variation in each one puts emphasis on a different group of muscles.

6. *Pulling springs apart.* Stand with feet together; raise the elbows so that fists are together, level with the chest. Slowly move fists apart, imagining you are with great difficulty pulling open a very heavy spring, and putting the stress on the muscles of the chest.

Asanas for firming and developing the bust:
Bow (page 142); Cobra (page 142); Head of a Cow (page 153).

To flatten the stomach, strengthen abdominal muscles and reduce fat

1. Standing with feet slightly apart, tense abdominal muscles until they are quite hard, then relax. Tense and relax . . . tense and relax . . . tense and relax.
2. With feet slightly apart, bend down and pick up an imaginary heavy bar, putting stress on the stomach muscles as you lift it. Repeat several times, relaxing between each movement.
3. Standing with feet apart, arms stretched forward with fists closed. Move the arms apart, as though pulling open a heavy spring, at the same time leaning backwards with the stress on stomach muscles. Repeat.
4. Standing with feet together, stretch arms in front and grasp an imaginary heavy bar. Raise it above head, keeping arms stiff and leaning backwards with stress on stomach and waistline muscles.
5. On the back, half lying, half reclining, with weight resting on bent elbows and legs stretched straight;

slowly raise and lower legs alternately, in a scissors movement, keeping knees straight and feeling the pull on the abdominal muscles. Repeat until slightly tired, then relax.

6. In the same position perform scissors movements of legs horizontally, to and from sides, crossing and recrossing legs. Repeat until slightly tired.

7. In same position separate legs and lift them, bringing them outwards, upwards and downwards in a circling movement. Repeat until slightly tired.

8. Sitting up with knees bent and level with shoulders, bend forward, stretching arms forward between knees and then pull back, in a rowing movement, stretching legs at the same time and putting tension on stomach muscles.

9. Lying on the back, raise the knees to the stomach, inhaling at the same time. Stretch legs up straight, lower them exhaling and relax. Repeat.

10. Lying with the knees up and feet flat on the floor. Inhale, sit up at same time stretching legs up, supporting yourself with palms flat on the floor by the sides. Lie back and relax. Repeat.

11. Lying on back with hands on waistline. Using alternate legs, kick up one leg, keeping it straight, then kick higher and at same time sit up without the help of the hands. Lie back and relax briefly before repeating action with other leg.

12. Sitting with both legs bent to left side and arms folded on chest. Stretch out both legs to the front,

then draw them in again to the right side, then to the front, then to the left, kicking them out and bringing them back in a continuous movement and trying not to lose your balance in the process.

13. Sitting with legs stretched out in front and arms folded on chest; swing the whole body over to the left, keeping it stiff and arching the back, then sit up again quickly in original position; swing over to right then sit up; repeat in continuous action, feeling stress on stomach muscles.

Asanas affecting the stomach muscles:
Cobra (page 142); Locust (page 143); Bow (page 142); Spinal Twist (page 141); Archer (page 140); all forward stretching *asanas* (page 137); Head-to-knee Pose (page 139); Supine Pelvic Pose (page 145); Plough (page 139); *Uddiyana* (page 149) and *Nauli* (page 150).

To firm and slim the waistline

1. With the left arm hanging by the side, lean slightly to the left and lift the right hand, bringing it up slowly, close to the side, with elbow bent and fist clenched as though lifting a heavy weight. Bring clenched fist right up into the armpit, stretching the muscles of the waistline, then lower the arm and let it hang by the side while you repeat the movement on the other side. Repeat several times slowly on each side, putting a strong pull on the muscles of the waist, and letting

the clenched fist almost brush the side as you raise it.
2. With left arm hanging, raise right arm sideways but this time keep it fully extended. Bring it up slowly as though lifting a heavy weight and putting stress on waist. Lower arm and repeat on other side. Repeat several times on each side.
3. Standing with feet apart, arms stretched forward with fists closed. Move the arms apart, as though pulling open a heavy spring, at the same time turning the body to the right. Face forward again with arms extended in front repeat the pulling-open movement, this time turning body to the left. Repeat each side four times, in a continuous movement. Be sure you do not twist the hips in turning. The twisting must be at the waistline only.
4. In the same position, with arms forward, this time lean back as you pull the spring open, feeling the tension in waistline and stomach.
5. With arms in front, grasp an imaginary heavy bar and raise it, keeping the arms stiff, and leaning backward with the stress on stomach and waistline muscles.
6. Standing with feet apart, raise the arms and join them overhead. Keeping the body straight, lean to the left, then up, to the right, then up; lower arms. Repeat four times but be sure you are bending only from the waistline and the upper part of the body is not bent forward.
7. In the same position, with the hands joined above the head, twist the upper part of the body, from waistline only, to left, then to right, keeping the soles of

the feet flat on the floor. Repeat four times.

8. See exercise number 12, for the stomach muscles, on page 160.

Asanas for the waistline:
Sideways swing (page 141); Twist (page 141); Head-to-knee (page 139); Stretching cycle (page 137).

To firm and slim the hips

1. Lying on the back, draw the knees up and keeping the soles of the feet flat on the floor move the legs and hips from side to side, keeping the upper body motionless. This movement must be adapted for individual requirements, for its purpose is to massage fat from the hips and buttocks. Each woman must decide for herself the point at which she needs to reduce and put the greatest weight on that particular spot in moving the legs from side to side.

2. Lying on the back with legs stretched out, link the arms on top of the head or fold them on the chest—anywhere so that they do not touch the ground. Keeping the body quite stiff, roll over to the left, arching your back as you go, so that you are pivoting with all your weight on the side of the hip; then roll over to the left side, repeating the arching movement. The purpose of the arching is to get the maximum weight on the hip and increase the effect of the massage.

3. Sitting down with legs stretched in front and hand on hips, thrust legs and hips forward alternately,

actually walking forward on buttocks. Then in the same way walk backwards.

4. See exercise number 12, for the stomach, on page 160.

5. Sitting with legs stretched out in front and arms folded on the chest, swing the stiffened body, stretched at full length, over to the left, taking all the weight on the left hip and arching the back; then sit up again quickly in original position—without any help from the hands—and swing over to the right and sit up. . . . Repeat four times in a continuous movement. This is the same exercise as number 13 on page 161, for the stomach, but this time the attention is concentrated on putting the body's weight on the hips.

6. Half lying, half reclining, with weight resting on elbows, raise right leg, bend the knee and perform an outward-circling movement, several times, stretching leg and pointing toe, and bringing leg back into position alongside the left leg; then repeat the movement with the left leg, getting good movement at the hips. Repeat four times on each side.

Asanas for the hips:

Spinal Twist (page 141); Sideways Swing (page 141); Archer (page 140); Bow (page 142); Plough (page 139); Head-to-knee (page 139); all cross-legged positions.

For improving and firming legs, thighs and calves

1. Standing with feet together, slowly rise up on the

toes; hold the position then come down and relax. Repeat four times.

2. Standing with feet together, rise up on toes, then slowly come down into a squatting position, with knees apart and back kept straight. Rise up slowly to standing position again and relax. Repeat four times.

3. Standing with feet together, move only toes, raising and lowering them all together, with the soles of the feet kept flat on the floor.

4. Standing with legs apart and hands on hips. Keep soles flat on the floor, bring knees in together until they touch, then apart, together-apart; together-apart. (For thighs.)

5. With feet apart and hands on hips. Bend the knees and come down into a half-squatting position, rising and coming down in a continuous, slightly springy movement.

6. With feet apart, heels flat on the floor, arms stretched forward and parallel. Slowly come down into a squatting position, making sure that the heels remain flat on the floor. Rise up and repeat four to six times.

7. With feet together and hands on hips, raise the right knee until the thigh is at right angles with the body, then stretch the lower leg and move it back and forth, each time trying to raise it a little higher. The thigh should be in the same position throughout. Change legs and repeat. (For thighs.)

8. Standing with legs together, raise right foot and

perform circular movement with ankle, first to the right, then to the left. Repeat with left ankle.
9. In same position, raise foot and move it up and down, up and down. Change sides and repeat.

Asanas for thighs and calves:
Bow (page 142); Locust (page 143); Supine Pelvic (page 145); Eagle Pose (page 152).

For arms, shoulders and back
For biceps and triceps. To prevent flabby upper arms
1. Standing straight, with arms by side, bend elbows and bring both hands up and forward in a scooping movement, flexing the biceps. When hands are about level with the waist, turn the wrists down, inwards and outwards in a circular movement and lower the arms. Repeat four times.
2. Standing with the arms outstretched at sides and palms facing upwards, turn the palms downwards and towards the back, so that the whole arm is turned. Continue the turning movement until the palms are facing up again, then reverse and turn them forward and upwards so that palms and arms are in original position. Repeat four times.

For shoulders and back
1. Bend the elbows and raise hands to level of the shoulders, so that the arms form a V on each side of the chest. Push the arms out sideways, pressing downwards, outwards and upwards in an undulating move-

ment, as though flying, squeezing and relaxing the spine and between the shoulder-blades with each movement.

2. The same position, but this time push out straight from the shoulders, not in an undulating movement.

3. With arms stretched out at sides, raise them up over the head, tensing as you raise them, then lower to shoulder-level again, making sure that the palms are facing downwards throughout the movement.

4. Stretch arms out straight at sides, level with shoulders, then rotate them in small circles, first in a forward movement, then in a backward direction. It is important not to bend the elbows. Repeat until slight tiredness in shoulders.

5. Bend the elbows and raise the arms with clenched fists close together in front of the chest. Slowly move the fists apart and back, as though opening a heavy spring, putting pressure on the spine and thus flushing the roots of the spinal nerves. Repeat four times.

6. With arms bent and fingertips on shoulders, bring elbows together in front of chest, then back to sides again, together, apart, together, apart.

12

Face, neck, and eye exercises

The face is made up of muscles which need exercising like any other part of the body, but which they rarely get in the ordinary course of modern life. In the days when people tore their food with their teeth the jaw and facial muscles received regular exercise and consequently a regular supply of blood, but the food we eat now is so soft that no effort is required to consume it. Mastication has been reduced to a minimum, which is not only bad for the teeth and gums but encourages unused facial muscles to grow flabby and to atrophy.

Apart from diet, rest and the general toning-up of the system, there are two different ways of benefiting the skin, tissues and muscles of the face: through facial exercises, and through the practice of positions that send an extra supply of blood to the face. Both should be done regularly.

Exercises

These should be practised before a mirror, until a slight tiredness is felt. The constructive power of the mind must be used and the thought held that you are going to achieve your objective.

1. Tense and relax the cheek muscles, slightly puffing out the cheeks, with lips compressed.
2. Open and close the mouth, with the lips forming the letter O.
3. Move the lower jaw from side to side.
4. Move the skin of the scalp backwards and forwards.

Asanas

The following poses stimulate the circulation in the face, feed the facial tissues and prevent and destroy wrinkles.

1. *Yoga-mudra*

If possible lock the legs in the Lotus position, otherwise sit in simple cross-legged pose. Clasp the hands behind the back, inhale and while exhaling bend forward and touch the floor with your forehead. With forehead still on the floor, inhale another breath and hold it for about five seconds until you feel the blood coming up into your face. Then rise up, exhale and pat the face briskly. This is a variation of *Yoga-mudra* (page 154), used for toning-up the face.

2. *Pose of a Child*

Sit back on your heels. Inhale, and as you exhale lean forward until your forehead is on the floor. Let your arms lie quite limply along each side of your bent legs. With forehead on the floor, inhale and hold the breath as long as you can, or until the blood comes to the face. Rise up, exhale and pat the face, as above. This is also a variation of a pose (see page 154) specially adapted for the facial tissues.

3. *Head of a Cow Pose*
Sitting on heels, bend arms behind the back so that you can grip hands together in region of the shoulder-blades. Inhale, exhale and bend forward. Inhale again, holding pose with forehead on floor until blood comes to the face, then rise up, exhale and pat the skin of the face (also a variation) (page 153).

4. *Stretching cycle*
Any of the forward-stretching *asanas* can be used to benefit the face by adapting the same method as described in the three poses above. After exhaling the breath, inhale again with the head held down on the knee, and hold the breath. Then come up, exhale and massage the face. (Page 137.)

5. *Pressing knees to stomach*
Lie on the back, bend the knees and while inhaling slowly bring them up and press to the stomach, using the hands to effect pressure. Hold the position until you feel the blood flooding into the face, then exhale and straighten out the legs, lowering them slowly to the floor. (This *asana* is also beneficial for flatulence and for strengthening stomach muscles.)

All the inverted poses, Headstand (page 135), Shoulderstand (page 131), Half-shoulderstand (page 133), should be practised regularly, particularly Half-shoulderstand. The raised poses, Bird (page 146) and Raven (page 147), are also instrumental in sending extra blood to the face.

See also the mental exercises on pages 48–52 and 100–104, which affect the face through the development and expression of inner peace and serenity.

Neck exercises

Practise each movement four times, moving only head and neck.

1. Raise and lower the head.
2. Turn the head from left to right and from right to left.
3. Slant the head towards the left shoulder, then to the right.
4. Raise the head, then let it fall forward on the chest. It should fall, not be lowered.
5. Push the chin out and draw it in again. (Anti-double-chin exercise.)
6. Rotate the head in a half-circle, to the right, drop the head to the chest, then rotate in a half-circle to the left.
7. Rotate the head in a complete circle, to the left, then to the right.

With hands clasped on the back of the neck, press the head down and forward, resisting with the neck.

Massage cheeks, forehead and nape of the neck by tapping with fingers.

Asanas which improve the neck include Pose of a Fish (page 143); Pose of a Camel (page 155); Cobra (page 142); Bow (page 142), and Head Pose (page 135).

Eye exercises

These eye exercises, practised regularly, are of the greatest importance in curing eye troubles or defective vision caused by muscular weakness. Women who suspect their sight is starting to decline should seriously consider improving the condition by exercise before going into glasses, which, though easier than regular exercising, can result only in weaker and weaker eyes.

Moving only the eyes, and each time trying to focus upon some point:

↑

1. Eyes up, down; up, down; up, down; close.

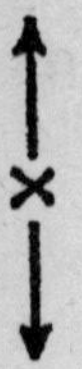

↓

↑
×
↓

2. Eyes up, straight ahead, down, straight ahead, up, straight ahead, down, straight ahead, up, straight ahead, down, straight ahead, close.

3. Eyes left, right; left, right; left, right; close.

4. Eyes left, straight ahead, right, straight ahead, left, straight ahead, right, straight ahead, left, straight ahead, right, straight ahead, close.

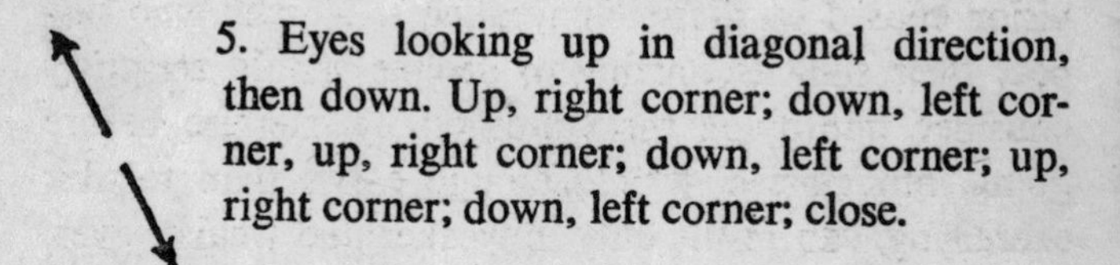

5. Eyes looking up in diagonal direction, then down. Up, right corner; down, left corner, up, right corner; down, left corner; up, right corner; down, left corner; close.

6. Change . . . up, left corner, down right corner . . . etc. Close.

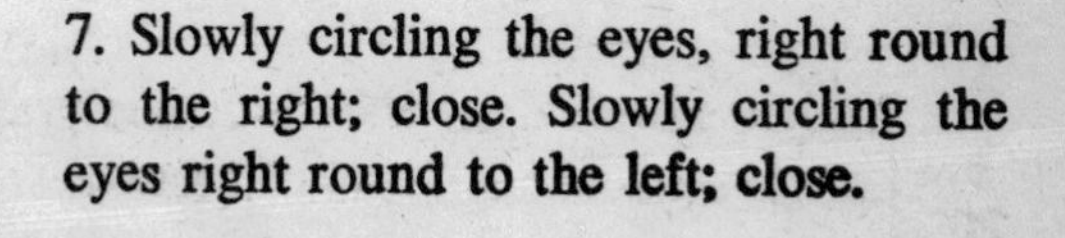

7. Slowly circling the eyes, right round to the right; close. Slowly circling the eyes right round to the left; close.

Changing of focus:

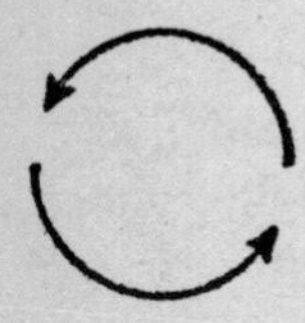

8. Look at the tip of your nose, then at a point in the distance; nose, distance, nose, distance; close.

9. Look at the tip of your finger, held about a foot away, then at the distance; finger, distance; finger, distance; close.

10. Practise looking at an object without blinking . . . not staring in the sense of straining but trying to see it more clearly.

11. Massage the eyes by squeezing the lids tightly together, then blinking rapidly several times.

12. Practise palming . . . placing the palms of the hands over the eyes to completely exclude the light.

APPENDIX I

Yoga and natural childbirth

Pregnancy and childbirth are not illnesses, they are natural physical functions which, like other physical activities, make certain demands on the body. The old idea that a pregnant woman was an invalid is now replaced by the far more sensible one of putting her into training, as though preparing for a contest of strength. Bringing a child into the world is a strenuous affair; it is hard physical labour—hence its name—so it stands to reason that women in good physical condition will acquit themselves better than those with flabby muscles and weak powers of endurance.

In many cities ante-natal classes are now held to teach pregnant women exercises that will help them in giving birth, but even without these specific exercises a woman who has practised yoga for some time will find the experience much easier than she would otherwise, provided of course that there are no physical defects or abnormalities to cause complications. Her muscles are flexible and controlled, her whole system toned-up, her general health good; she knows how to relax her body, nerves and mind, she understands breath control and how to re-charge and replenish expended vitality. She approaches childbirth as a trained athlete approaches a contest, calmly and with confidence, knowing that everything is in her favour; and after the event she quickly recovers her strength, her figure and her *joie de vivre.*

Led by pioneering obstetricians, increasing numbers of women are now practising for so-called natural childbirth, training themselves by exercises, deep breathing and relaxation techniques, and helping to regain their figures by post-natal exercises. Women who have practised both yoga and natural childbirth often remark that a number of the exercises are the same, and this is true; in fact, some of the pregnancy exercises are almost identical with yoga exercises. There are, of course, variations for certain purposes . . . for example breathing through the mouth (panting) is taught for use during the actual delivery, but in general there is a great resemblance.

If you are a yoga student, wishing to prepare for childbirth but for some reason unable to attend ante-natal classes, you could, with your doctor's approval, achieve almost the same results by concentrating on certain yoga techniques and exercises. These will not of course give you instructions for actual childbirth procedure but will prepare your nerves and muscles in exactly the same way as the ante-natal exercises.

After the third month it is advisable to give up most of the usual *asanas*—though some women continue to practise inverted poses, apart from Headstand, and forward-stretching movements until the sixth or seventh month; but in any case nothing should be done without the doctor's consent, and no exercises attempted that involve strenuous upward stretching, violent stomach contractions or anything that might adversely affect the position of the child. The Head-stand is forbidden for this reason.

Ante-natal exercises

Relaxation. Practise *Savasana,* as described on page 117, and learn to relax at will your muscles, nerves and mind. Starting with the tips of the toes, relax all the groups of muscles, including the face, arms and hands; then withdraw nervous energy, establish deep breathing and finally send your mind right away and practise complete detachment.

Breathing. Practise your breathing exercises regularly (pages 124–7) night and morning if you can, with special attention to cycles involving retention of breath.

Cross-legged positions. All the cross-legged poses are beneficial to pregnant women. If possible lock your legs in the Lotus position; otherwise practise any of the other poses . . . half-Lotus, Position of an Adept or Free Pose. Position of a Hero could also be included. The poses help to loosen the hips and stretch the muscles of the pelvic floor.

Squatting. With feet slightly apart and parallel, try to squat down, keeping soles and heels flat on the floor. This is difficult at first, and it will help if you keep your arms stretched out before you, with one hand clasping the wrist of the other.

Contraction of muscles. Practise *Aswini-mudra,* as described on page 154. This can be done lying flat on the back as well as in a sitting position.

Pose of a Cat. Kneeling, with hands on the floor and arms straight, head hanging down, manipulate the spine by raising it up and then letting it go slack, forming a hump in the back, then a deep depression (Plate 23). The name of the exercise comes from the movement of a cat when flexing and relaxing its spine.

Lying on the back, press the back to the floor, then arch it, still keeping hips and shoulders on the floor.

Lying on the back, with knees bent and feet flat on the floor, move bent legs from side to side, exercising muscles in the waist.

Post-natal exercises

To help regain your figure after the child is born practise all the above exercises, gradually adding to them, with your doctor's consent, until you are able to return to normal yoga practice. Relaxation could be done lying flat on the stomach with arms limply by the sides, while still in bed, and also in bed you could practise arching and relaxing the back, with the following variations:

1. Lying on the back, inhale and raise chest only; exhale and relax.
2. Inhale and raise hips only; exhale and relax.

3. Inhale and raise head only; exhale and relax.

You could also exercise the feet and ankles while still in bed, tensing and relaxing the toes, and moving the feet up and down, at the ankle joint, and round in a circular movement.

When out of bed again consult your doctor, and if he approves try exercises given in Chapter 11 for regaining firmness of breasts and slimness of stomach and waistline. Supplement them with the following exercises, designed to regain strong abdominal muscles:

1. Lie flat on the back. Inhale and slowly raise both legs up to an angle of 45 degrees. Exhale. Lower legs. Repeat four to six times.
2. With hands under the neck, inhale and slightly raise head and shoulders. Exhale and relax.
3. Lie flat on the back with arms stretched over the head. Inhale, stretch the body, feeling a gentle pull in the abdominal muscles. Relax, exhaling, swing arms forward and sit up. Then lie down again and repeat.
4. Reclining on the forearms, inhale, drawing knees to the chest, stretch legs up, exhale and lower legs to the floor. Repeat four to six times.
5. Lying flat on the back with hands on the waistline, inhale, raise head and shoulders, and legs, to equal height, contracting abdominal muscles. Relax.
6. Lying flat on the back, with knees to the stomach. Inhale and stretch legs vertically up. Exhale, drop legs back to the stomach. Relax.

7. Reclining on the forearms, breathing freely, draw both knees to the stomach, swing them to the right in a circular movement, stretching the legs as they near the floor. Make a complete circle to the other side, draw them back to the stomach and then repeat the circle. Practise two or three times to the right, two or three times to the left. Relax. (In this exercise not only the abdominal muscles are strengthened but the waistline is firmed and slimmed.)

APPENDIX II

Practising at home

Students often ask what they should do about practice; if it is necessary to practise every day and for how long? What are the most important exercises to do and how many should be done at a time? When is the best time of day to practise, and so on.

The first of these questions is the only one which has the same answer for everyone. If you really want to make progress and get the fullest benefit from physical yoga you should practise every day, preferably always at the same time, so that the body, trained to expect its toning-up at regular intervals, can best respond to it. Try to find or *make* the time needed, taking it from something else if necessary, which is what busy people usually have to do; but if your time is not your own and daily practice is really impossible, do the best you can, trying to do some *asanas* at least several times a week.

It may be easier to do your practising in sections rather than in one uninterrupted sequence, though this of course is the best arrangement. A busy housewife with children could, for example, do some breathing exercises when she first gets up, and if there is time a few of the slow movements, for the bust or waistline. Stomach contractions could be done under the shower, and then when the children have gone to school, the baby is asleep, breakfast is digested and most of the housework done, she could devote half an hour, just before lunch, to as many of the *asanas* and exercises as she can. This time—about midday—is the best for most women at home, for if they leave it until later they must wait until lunch has been digested, then there will probably be children coming home from school and after that dinner to prepare. If a determined effort is made to set aside that half-hour before lunch and let nothing interfere with it, it will become quite automatic and the body will actually look forward to it.

Always start with a few minutes of relaxation, to prepare body and mind for what is to come; then do some limbering-up, to warm-up the muscles; then the breathing cycles. After this the inverted poses should come, followed by neck and eye exercises, the stretching cycles and finally, after further relaxation, the Headstand and any raised poses. This order of exercises is the traditional pattern of instruction practised in the east and is the most logical sequence to follow.

Remember that breathing is always done through the nose, unless exhalation through the mouth is mentioned.

Do not worry if at first you cannot remember all the poses or exercises. Do the ones you can remember.

The others will become quite familiar with time.

Yoga should never be practised on a full stomach, and after a heavy meal at least three hours should be allowed to pass before exercises are done. Stomach contractions should be done only on a completely empty stomach and never during menstruation or in pregnancy. During menstruation do not practise anything that causes discomfort or distress. Concentrate on breathing and relaxation at these times.

In the general practice of the *asanas* the student is expected to use her common sense, eliminating anything that she knows is unsuitable for her, and concentrating on those that she needs the most. In the body-moulding cycles she should decide which part of her figure needs greatest improvement and should select and concentrate on the appropriate exercises; but she should not neglect her general condition and should try to keep up a regular practice of most of the important *asanas*.

Apart from those included specifically for improving women's figures, the poses and exercises given in this book form the nucleus of physical yoga and if they are all practised the body will receive all-over development and benefit.

Remember that any exercise affecting different sides of the body must be done on both left and right sides, otherwise there will be uneven development.

If there is really not time to practise more than a couple of exercises or positions and a choice must be made the best thing is to determine which you need most . . . for instance, if your nerves are bad you will give priority to relaxation and breathing; if you have thyroid deficiency, are overweight, or suffer from sexual debility concentrate on the Shoulderstand, and so on; but if you have no particular problem and are seeking only a general improvement, try always to include some deep breathing, the stomach contractions, relaxation and the Shoulderstand. Add other exercises according to the time at your disposal.

Do your exercises on a rug, mat or folded blanket, or a foam-rubber mat, anything that is comfortable. Do not practise to a state of exhaustion and remember to rest and relax between each *asana*. After finishing the Headstand or the inverted poses lie quietly for a minute to allow your circulation to return to normal. Try to shut out telephones and doorbells while you are practising and impress on your family that you must not be disturbed for trivial reasons. This short period once a day is the least you are entitled to and should be kept exclusively for yourself and your self-improvement.

Some people say they can only find time to practise in the early morning, by getting up earlier. For some exercises, such as breathing, this is the best time of the day and yogis believe that the air and the sun's rays at this time are specially full of *prana*; but often the body is stiff after the night's sleep and it may be difficult to do positions that can be done easily later in the day when the muscles have been warmed-up by moving about. The evening, before eating, is a good time, but is not always a convenient time for women who must be cooking meals or feeding children, and if they leave their practice until after dinner they must wait until the meal has been digested and then it may be inconvenient from social or family points of view. Don't be persuaded to demonstrate yoga at parties, It is quite likely that as soon as your friends know you are a student they will want you to stand on your head. This seems to be inevitable in many cases, but do not co-operate. Yoga is not a side-show or a circus stunt for entertaining bystanders, and it can also be very dangerous if performed at parties, for the chances are that you will have been eating or drinking or both, which could cause drastic consequences.

Yoga should be learnt from a teacher, whenever possible, but if you live in a remote area where it is quite impossible to get personal instruction, be very cautious how you proceed if you are trying to learn from a book. A mis-reading or misunderstanding of an instruction could do damage and even cause an injury, and you should remember that nothing should ever be forced or strained. If you cannot do an *asana* at first do not push yourself . . . wait until your body is stronger and your muscles have become more elastic, as they will with regular practice. Try the positions, no matter how badly, with the idea of improving even a fraction more each day, no matter how long it takes. Eventually you will achieve your objective.

Be sure also that you have medical approval before

embarking on physical yoga, that there is nothing to forbid you doing certain positions such as the Headstand. It is true that such things as high blood-pressure and heart conditions can be improved by yoga breathing and relaxation, but it is best to make quite sure that you are taking no risks in practising any other *asanas*.

Try always to practise in the same place, if possible setting aside a room where you can relax, secure in the knowledge that people are not going to rush in and interrupt you or make you feel self-conscious by staring or asking questions. If you have a secluded garden or know a quiet beach or field where you will not be observed or interrupted, it is best of all to practise in the open, wearing a minimum of clothes; but wherever you practise remember that this time is *your* time, dedicated to yourself, your health, beauty and happiness.

TABLE OF ASANAS

* Denotes most important exercises for particular disorders

Conditions needing improvement	*Asanas or exercises recommended*
Asthma	Breathing with abdomen; Headstand; Fish; Shoulderstand; Locust; *Savasana.*
Backache	Cobra; Fish; Head of a Cow; Supine Pelvic.
Bust— to correct sagging to develop and firm	Bow; Cobra; Head of a Cow; Slow movements and exercises in Chapter 11.
Chin— to prevent double chin	Fish; Camel; Exercises in Chapter 12.
Constipation	Locust; Cobra; *Uddiyana*; *Nauli*; Fish; Lotus; Headstand; Shoulderstand; Half-shoulderstand; Archer; Spinal Twist; *Yoga-mudra*; Supine Pelvic; Head-to-knee, sitting and standing.
Digestive troubles including flatulence*	*Uddiyana*; *Nauli*; Lotus; Headstand; Shoulderstand; Half-shoulderstand; Plough; Spinal Twist; Head-to-knee; Supine Pelvic; Locust;* Cobra;* Bow;* Wheel;* Archer; Knees pressed to stomach—pages 42–3.*
Excess weight	Wheel; Head-to-knee; Shoulderstand; Plough; Bow; Arch Gesture; Spinal Twist; *Uddiyana.*
Hips—to reduce fat	Archer; Twist; Bow; Sideways swing; Plough; Head-to-knee; Exercises in Chapter 11.

Lack of poise	Tree; Eagle; Lotus.
confidence	Spinal twist; Cobra; Lotus; Headstand.
concentration	Headstand.
sleep	Triangular; Rocking; Plough; Locust; Head-to-knee; *Savasana*; Breathing cycles.
relaxation	*Savasana*; Breathing cycles.
inner strength imagination courage will-power	Pose of a hero; Mental exercises described in Chapter 3 and Chapter 6.
energy	Headstand; Shoulderstand; Bow; Wheel; Head-to-knee; Spinal Twist; Bird; Raven; Re-charging exercises in Chapter 3.
Menopause disorders	Bow; Cobra; Shoulderstand; Fish; Plough; Locust; Head-to-knee; Headstand; *Uddiyana*; *Nauli*.
Menstrual disorders	Bow; Cobra; Shoulderstand; Fish; Plough; Locust; Headstand; *Uddiyana*; *Nauli*; Head-to-knee, sitting and standing.
Nervous conditions, including fatigue, bad memory, depression	Headstand; Shoulderstand; Locust; Bow; *Savasana*; Head-to-knee; Mental exercises in Chapter 6.
Ovarian insufficiency	Shoulderstand; Fish; Cobra; Locust; Half-shoulderstand; Headstand; Wheel; *Nauli*; Head-to-knee.
Premature ageing	Headstand; Shoulderstand; Half-shoulderstand; *Uddiyana*; *Nauli*; Physical and mental exercises in Chapter 3. Slow movements in Chapter 11.
Prolapse	Headstand; Shoulderstand; Half-shoulderstand; *Uddiyana*.
Puberty disorders	Shoulderstand; Fish; Plough; Cobra; Locust; Head-to-knee, sitting and standing.

TABLE OF ASANAS

Respiratory troubles	Locust; Fish; Breathing cycles; *Savasana*.
Sexual debility, including Sterility*	Shoulderstand; Half-shoulderstand; Headstand;* Bow;* Head-to-knee; Plough; Fish; Supine Pelvic; Eagle;* Spinal Twist; *Aswini-mudra*; *Uddiyana*. See also Chapter 4.
Spinal stiffness	Spinal twist; Bow; Arch Gesture; Knee-to-head; Archer; Candle; Plough; Cobra; Locust; Head of a Cow; Stretching cycles.
Stomach—sagging to remove fat	Shoulderstand; Half-shoulderstand; Bow;* *Uddiyana*;* *Nauli*;* Archer;* Twist;* Plough;* Lotus; Head-to-knee;* Exercises in Chapter 11.*
Thighs—to firm and improve	Supine Pelvic; Bow; Locust; Exercises in Chapter 11.
Thyroid deficiency	Shoulderstand; Bow; Plough; Cobra; Locust; Head-to-knee.
Uterine disorders, including catarrh of the uterus	Shoulderstand; Headstand; Locust.
Varicose veins	All inverted poses, including Headstand.
Waistline—to reduce and firm	Sideways swing; Spinal Twist; Stretching cycle; Exercises in Chapter 11.
Wrinkles	Half-shoulderstand; Headstand; *Yoga-mudra*; Head of a Cow; Pose of Child; Facial exercise in Chapter 12.

NAMES OF ASANAS

English	*Sanscrit*
Easy Pose (cross-legged)	Sukhasana
Pose of an Adept	Siddhasana
Half-Lotus	Ardha-Padmasana
Lotus	Padmasana
Free Pose	Samasana
Pose of a Hero	Virasana
Pose of Complete Rest	Savasana
Shoulderstand	Sarvangasana
Half-shoulderstand	Vipareeta-karani
Choking Pose	Karnapeetasana
Headstand	Sirshasana
Locked Headstand (legs in Lotus position)	Oordhva padmasana
Arch Gesture	Janusirasana
Head-to-knee: Sitting	Paschimatanasana
Standing	Padahastasana
Plough	Halasana
Archer	Akarshana Dhanurasana
Spinal Twist	Ardha-matsyendrasana
Cobra	Bhujangasana
Bow	Dhanurasana
Locust	Salabhasana
Fish	Matsyasana
Wheel	Chakrasana
Supine Pelvic	Supta-Vajrasana

Pose of a Raven	Kakasana
Stomach contractions	Uddiyana
Separation of recti muscles	Nauli
Tree (balancing)	Vkrasana
Eagle	Garudasana
Head of a Cow Pose	Gomukhasana
Pose of a Camel	Ushtrasana